FOOD ISN'T MEDICINE

FOOD ISN'T MEDICINE

HOW MISINFORMATION IS HARMING OUR HEALTH

DR JOSHUA WOLRICH

BSc (Hons) MBBS MRCS ANutr

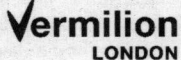

Vermilion
LONDON

Vermilion, an imprint of Ebury Publishing,
20 Vauxhall Bridge Road,
London SW1V 2SA

Vermilion is part of the Penguin Random House group of companies
whose addresses can be found at global.penguinrandomhouse.com

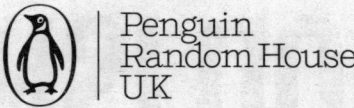

Penguin
Random House
UK

First published by Vermilion in 2021
This edition published by Vermilion in 2022

www.penguin.co.uk

A CIP catalogue record for this book is available from the British Library

ISBN 9781785043468

Printed and bound in Great Britain by Clays Ltd, Elcograf S.p.A.

The authorised representative in the EEA is Penguin Random House Ireland,
Morrison Chambers, 32 Nassau Street, Dublin D02 YH68

Penguin Random House is committed to
a sustainable future for our business, our readers
and our planet. This book is made from Forest
Stewardship Council® certified paper.

For those experiencing weight stigma:
please know you deserve so much better and
I promise not to stop until you get it.

CONTENTS

PREFACE

'You are completely entitled to opinions that
are not supported by evidence, but the
moment you spread that opinion as fact, you
are a liar, and if you spread it as fact
knowing that it's not supported by evidence,
you are both a liar and a fraud.'

OCCAM'S BARBER

On the 16th of August 2020, Justin Bieber and I became friends.

Okay fine, he publicly told me to 'fuck off' for challenging him in front of his then 144 million Instagram followers, but that's basically the same thing, right? Friend, acquaintance, mortal enemy . . . what's the difference?!

I'll explain how that all came about in a second, but first let me introduce myself. I'm an NHS junior doctor currently in the middle of a postgraduate master's degree in nutrition. I've grown increasingly frustrated over the last few years seeing how some medical doctors have become bolder in believing that they understand nutritional science. Let's be clear right out of the gate; the scientific study of the relationship between diet and health is *not* the same discipline that we get taught in medical school, otherwise my current academic study would be a waste of money. Doctors are first and foremost biomedical scientists, meaning that we focus on learning how the human body functions in order to understand and treat disease. There's less overlap with nutrition

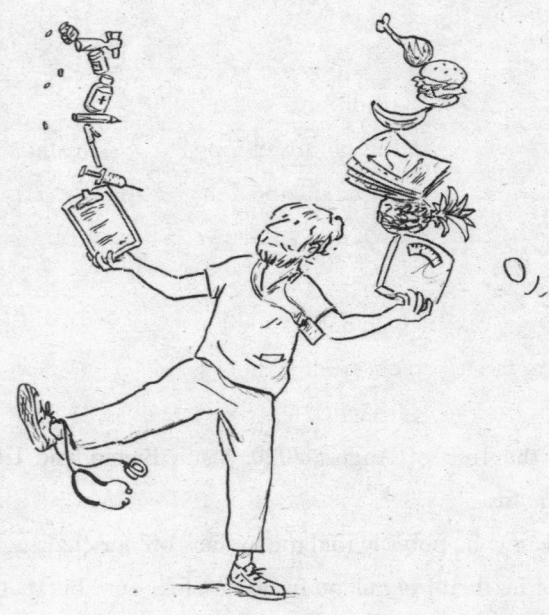

than you might immediately think and an ignorance of the fundamental differences between the two disciplines has resulted in a truly terrible slew of books being written and published by doctors way out of their lane.

Of the top 100 bestselling books on nutrition in 2018, guess which profession made up the biggest percentage of authorship? You are four times more likely to pick up a nutrition book written by a doctor than you would by a dietitian or nutritionist[1]. If this were the other way around and medical books were being overwhelmingly written by people without a medical degree, I can guarantee you that doctors would be up in arms.

Not only that, but the nutritional advice found in these books varies widely and is often completely contradictory. Eat carbs, don't eat carbs; eat fat, don't eat fat; go vegan, or is it carnivore?! They promise weight loss and disease cures. We've reached a point now where both traditional and social media are awash with so much nonsense that it's almost impossible for anyone to figure out what's actually true. Oh . . . and don't get me started on books that claim to explain why 'everything we've been told about food is wrong'. Burn them all.

Nutritional science actually knows an *incredible* amount about food and its impact on our health, but facts like 'eat more veg' aren't exactly sexy, are they? It's much more exciting for someone to claim they're 'challenging the status quo' and dogmatically promise a new solution to health and weight loss, even though those two categorically aren't even the same thing. We'll get to that.

Food Isn't Medicine

In my humble opinion there is one simple truth that I believe would solve a lot of the difficulty sifting through the misinformation when it comes to nutrition: *food isn't medicine**.

The vast majority of nutrition books rely on the opposite being true, despite the fact that you'd be hard-pressed to find anyone with formal training in dietetics or nutrition who uses the phrase. That alone should really tell you something.

The fact that food isn't medicine is not a bad thing by any means; it's actually a really *good* thing that it's not! Our health is

---

* I'm well aware that in the context of severe eating disorders recovery this phrase can be very useful, especially for those requiring inpatient treatment. I'm not here to invalidate that. This specific exception doesn't make the rule for the rest of us.

too often sold as something we have complete control over, and treating food as medicine only serves to encourage this rhetoric of personal responsibility. We need to stop shaming people for what they eat and implying that an illness was their fault for not making better choices.

Recognising that food isn't medicine doesn't mean I don't believe food can have a positive impact on someone's health – this isn't an either/or situation! Not only can the way we live our lives have a big impact on chronic disease, but helping people come off medication they believed to be lifelong is a wonderful aim. Ironically, accepting the differences between food and medicine leads to this pursuit becoming more realistic and attainable.

Hang on a second, didn't Hippocrates, the so-called 'father of Western medicine', say to 'let food be thy medicine and medicine be thy food'? Sorry to burst a bubble right at the beginning of this book but Hippocrates never actually combined the two; this is simply a nice-sounding misquote[2]. Although Hippocrates was ahead of his time back in 400 BC about many aspects of medicine, it's a little problematic to be using things that he said (or supposedly said) as instruction on how to practise it today. For example, he believed that you could stop someone having a period by applying 'as large a cupping instrument as possible to the breasts'[3] . . . but no one is quoting him on that one, are they?

This obsession with wanting food to be medicine has resulted in increasing numbers of doctors playing identity politics with their dietary choices. Their social media handles now include phrases like 'low-carb' or 'carnivore' as a badge of honour.

When diet infiltrates someone's identity it can all too often lead to bias and closed-mindedness. When shown evidence that puts this new part of who they are into question, do you really think they're going to take the time to genuinely explore it? We are all perfectly entitled to choose to eat a certain way, but as doctors we *have* to keep this from being projected onto patients during a consultation.

Back to Bieber

I'd come across a post that Justin had made on his Instagram with the words: 'The Right Healthy Food Is Actually Medicine'. The caption underneath doubled down and read: 'If you are feeling anxious or depressed a lot of it has to do with our diet! Try changing up your diet! It has helped me so much!!!' I had a feeling that the Beliebers wouldn't take kindly to me challenging him on his messaging, but I couldn't let something like that just exist without trying to add some nuance, especially when it was by someone with so much influence. I left the following comment underneath:

'The intention behind this post is good, but unfortunately the potential outcome is quite harmful. Food is many, many things but it's not medicine. That's not to say it isn't important – it provides us with nutrition and energy to thrive, but it has its limitations. Anxiety and depression are very rarely as a result of food intake. Mental health is complex and boiling it down to the privilege of food

choices is incorrect and stigmatising for those who
struggle with it on a daily basis. For any of you who read
this and felt a sense of guilt that if only you changed
your food you wouldn't struggle with mental health . . .
please know that's not accurate. You are doing a fantastic
job – do not compare yourself to a celebrity with all the
capacity for change and privilege in the world.'

My purpose here wasn't to specifically get Bieber's attention (it's
rarely ever about the original poster in these kinds of situations),
but instead to provide some reality to those members of the public
who might have read his post and been misled. What I couldn't
have predicted was the fact that he put my comment in his Instagram stories and said: 'Bro litterally [sic] fuck off lol'.

While fending off the subsequent slew of hate messages from
his followers I ended up chatting to him over direct message for
about an hour. He quoted the dictionary definition of medicine to
me (a common argument) and then claimed that food can 'heal
your frontal lobes' (a less common one). After quite a bit of back
and forth in which I said things such as, 'of course everything can
be taken out of context but that's not an excuse to ignore the
impact our words can have', I noticed that he'd actually changed
the caption on his post very slightly to add some nuance. Instead
of saying, 'If you are feeling anxious or depressed a lot of it has to
do with our diet', it now read, '. . . it can often have a lot to do
with our diet'. Movement in the right direction, however small, is
movement nonetheless.

The last thing he said to me was, 'the tone of my fuck off was meant to be cheeky not mean'. I'm taking that reassurance to imply we're now friends. My DMs are always open Justin.

Not another diet book

This book has been a labour of love and I really hope that you find it useful when navigating the current state of nutritional discourse. I want this to be an encyclopaedia of nutribollocks that you can refer back to time and time again after the first read through.

> **nutribollocks** /njʊˈtrɪbɒləks/
>
> *noun* VULGAR SLANG • BRITISH
>
> nonsense nutrition advice with little to no scientific
>   evidence; promotes disordered eating habits.
> 'drinking apple cider vinegar in order to lose weight is
>   complete nutribollocks'
>
> early 21st century: blend of nutrition and bollocks

I want to empower you to be able to filter through diet culture and come out the other side with a more relaxed view on nutrition and your health. I want you to be able to confidently challenge it not only when Katy Perry tells you to bathe in apple cider vinegar and Novak Djokovic tells you to drink celery juice, but when your best friend tells you about their new fasting regime that they want you to do with them. I want you to understand why the 'food is medicine' rhetoric is misguided so that you find it easier to avoid the nutribollocks it encourages.

There is a *lot* of nonsense that we could go through but I've

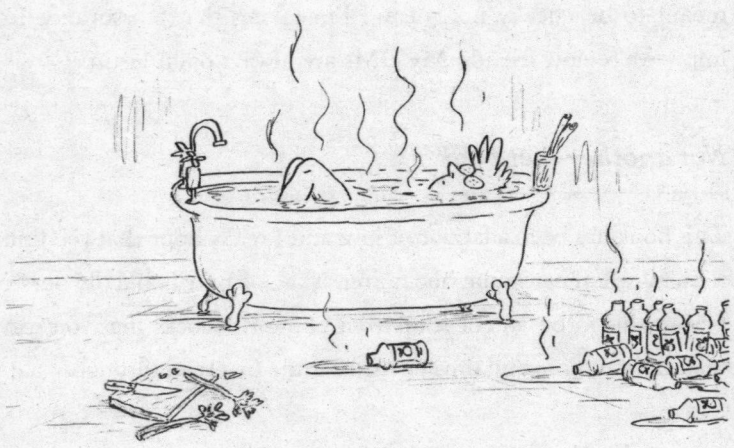

chosen the topics that I believe come up the most frequently, and also cover the most bases possible. To note, this *categorically isn't* a diet book claiming to show you how to lose weight. I'll explain why that's the case in the first couple of chapters.

I wish I had a book like this a few years ago when I was trying to sift through the conflicting information available online. Searching for answers on Google doesn't really help unless you know what you're looking for and it personally led me down a path of bro-science and bodybuilding forums. I started demonising carbs and buying books that proclaimed food was medicine, the latter of which now sit gathering dust on my bookshelf; I don't particularly want to regift them and risk someone else being misled. My hope is that this book either saves you from a similar fate or acts as a lifeline to help pull you out. Remember, there's absolutely no shame in changing your mind on something you thought was true.

Scientific cheat sheet

In order to address the nutribollocks in this book we need to have discussions about research and different types of scientific studies. I'm aware that academic language can mean very little to some, so to try to address that problem I wanted to include a cheat sheet of sorts right here at the beginning.

Hopefully this will be something you can refer back to if need be and should also serve you well for understanding more of what you come across online.

Anecdotes	Stories from personal testimony. This is the lowest form of scientific evidence as it is heavily influenced by things like bias. While that doesn't mean we should automatically disregard someone's experience as incorrect, it's incredibly important not to draw wider conclusions from it.
Association/ Correlation	A link between two things where one may or may not be as a result of the other.
Causation	A link between two things where one has been proven to be as a result of the other.
Cohort Study	A study following one group of people over a period of time, usually consisting of individuals who are at risk of developing a specific disease. Different behaviours and factors are noted throughout in order to investigate the cause of the disease if/when it occurs.
Case-control Study	A study comparing two groups of people, one with a condition and one without. They are usually retrospective, meaning that researchers look back in time to see if different factors can be identified between the groups.

Randomised Controlled Trial (RCT)	This is an experimental study where people are randomly assigned to two (or more) groups and then given different interventions. One of these groups is usually given a placebo to be able to compare against. This is often considered good quality evidence.
Metabolic Ward Study	This is a tightly controlled study where participants live full time at a research unit. They are monitored 24/7 with everything from food to exercise and sleep being controlled, measured and documented. If designed correctly these studies can be incredibly reliable.
Meta-analysis	This is a way of using statistics to combine the results of multiple studies to try to find if a conclusion can be drawn. This is useful as studies looking at the same topic can often show conflicting results when analysed individually.
Systematic Review	This is a review of all the available research on a particular subject. Studies that are of poor quality are often excluded. This is usually combined with a meta-analysis as the way of analysing the research.

1.

PRINGLES AND ICE CREAM

To give you some context as to how I became passionate about nutrition and challenging diet culture, it's probably best to start right at the beginning. The privilege of growing up in a household where I enjoyed home-cooked meals the majority of the time contributed to me gaining a love of food from an early age. My father had always cooked as a hobby, and after finding himself assuming the role of the stay-at-home dad, my two younger siblings and I could always count on an interesting evening meal from a multitude of different cuisines. How could disordered eating have reared its ugly head from that seemingly peachy situation?

After losing his mother to pneumonia and a brother to suicide within days of each other, my father's relationship with alcohol became even more challenging for us. My memory of the full timeline is a little hazy, but there are several things still vivid to this day; ones that I feel probably affected me more than my parents' subsequent divorce.

Food insecurity

As the years went on, evening mealtimes became increasingly difficult. Usually I'd get food, but my father's once impeccable judgement of appropriate spice levels went steadily out of the window. Punished if I didn't eat it, I grew a tolerance to chilli like no other child in my white, middle-class neighbourhood. Unpleasant as that was, it was still better than the other days when I'd be sent to bed without any food at all. Arguing never worked.

I decided that my only option was to have food stashed away so I didn't have to wait until my mother got home late from work to eat something. As a pre-teen child I wasn't exactly rolling in pocket money, so I resorted to slightly less legal ways of ensuring I didn't go hungry.

There was a corner shop on my walk home from school that I would frequent for sweets and the like. Of the two aisles in the store, the one furthest away from the counter had a blind spot that I may or may not have used to get really good at pretending to look for something in my backpack, while simultaneously knocking a full tub of Pringles off the shelf into it. I honestly can't believe I never got caught. I still feel guilty about it to this day but I'm happy to report that my brief stint as an accomplished thief didn't continue into adulthood (just to clarify).

Was the act of eating an entire tub of Pringles straight after school good for me? Probably not. Did my relationship with food take a hit during that period? Definitely. May it have even led to me overeating on a regular basis since I would still ask my mother for dinner when she got home? Sure. Is the act of eating when

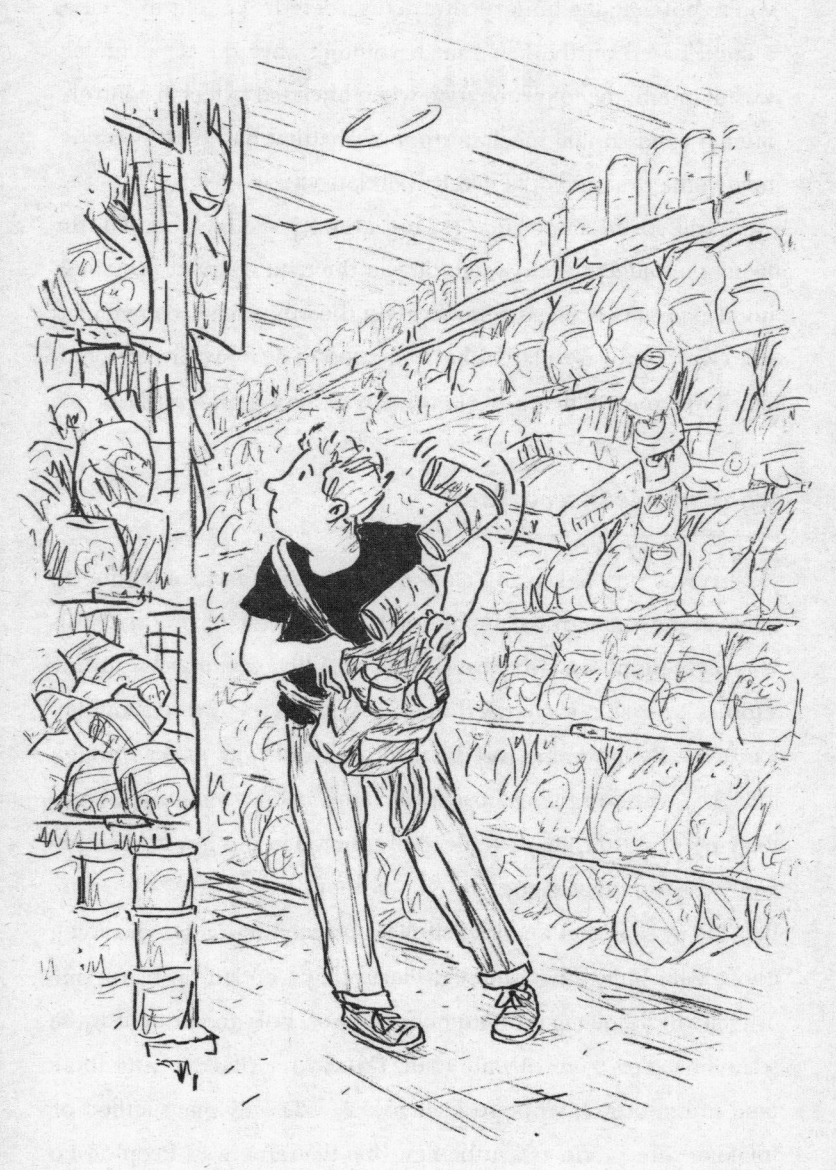

you're not actually hungry always disordered? No, but to do it as a child based on the fear that I wouldn't have dinner definitely was. It taught me to rely on food when I needed to feel in control – often a valid coping mechanism, but one that has great potential to become dysfunctional if relied on long-term.

I will spend some time talking about just how complex the factors influencing our weight are in the next chapter, but childhood experiences like the one I've just described likely contributed as to why I grew up a larger kid than most. The first time I remember it making a difference to my life was during junior school.

Body image insecurities

There was one kid in my class who always found something to pick on me about: my hair was too long or too short; my nose was too big; I didn't have any friends (or I had the wrong ones); or my clothes were shit. It changed weekly. At times the unpredictability became all-consuming as I tried to work out how to get through the day without giving him something new to bully me about. Having said that, there was one reason he could always consistently rely on: my weight.

There is always an element of insecurity and cowardice with those who bully. I'm ashamed to say that I ended up being one myself the following year after changing schools and both of those elements rang true with me then. I'd left one place feeling small and unimportant, while believing there was only one method of making sure I didn't start the new one the same way. People who abuse others for their size as adults are no different. Add in the anonymity of the internet and it can embolden those who may not dare to discriminate face to face.

From those early years, until relatively recently, I spent a large proportion of my life trying to lose weight. My worth as a human became intrinsically linked to what I looked like and the number on the scales; I had it in my head that I was neither attractive nor worthy of love unless I was slimmer. These same insecurities continued even when I was in my first long-term relationship and ended up playing a major role in its eventual breakdown. It made me a possessive partner, which, completely reasonably, resulted in being dumped. At the time, my lack of insight simply led to a doubling down on my weight-loss efforts in an attempt to be attractive enough not to be dumped again. Retrospect is a wonderful thing eh?

Being a doctor sounded cool

Growing up I had a real mixture of different career goals, from being a chess grandmaster or professional chef to being a singer. How different life would have been if I'd have succeeded in my audition for S Club Juniors! Despite doctor never featuring on that list, I came home from school at the age of 16 and told my mother that I was going to study medicine at university. The careers counsellor had been in that day and I remember being given this thick career book to pick from. The thought of being a teacher didn't sound fun as I knew how difficult my classmates and I could be; the broad title of scientist just made me think of working in a lab; but the last 'match' was doctor, which I thought sounded cool. I can still hear my mother's understandably sceptical response to this day, along with a raised eyebrow:

'We'll see.'

With no doctors in my immediate family, I arrived at medical school relatively naive as to what the job would bring. Being a doctor can be really emotionally draining, from fighting against the government on changing job contracts to working long hours during a pandemic without adequate protective equipment. It's not a job you would stick at unless you really loved it; I hope I continue to love it as much as I do now for the rest of my life.

Disordered eating

When I graduated from university, a different reason for wanting to lose weight emerged; I believed that I couldn't be a good doctor unless I was thinner. After the years of being stigmatised for my weight (both individually and on a societal level) I had unconsciously accepted the negative stereotypes onto myself. What I now recognise as internalised weight stigma led to me feeling an overwhelming sense of hypocrisy whenever I recommended weight loss to my patients, as I myself was labelled 'overweight' and therefore 'unhealthy'. I truly felt there was no way patients would take my health advice seriously – the analogy I'd used in my head was that of a stop-smoking service being run by a smoker. The comparison made sense to me at the time as I'd been taught weight was a lifestyle choice I simply hadn't been trying hard enough to change. We'll talk more about that in the next chapter.

I decided to create an Instagram account in 2016 with the sole intention of keeping me 'accountable' during my weight loss (a logical step as, let's be honest, that's what so much of Instagram is used for). I remember promising myself that if I ate a biscuit, I would post a picture of said biscuit; that way my friends would tell me off for eating it and I would eat fewer biscuits and stay 'strong' with my diet. First, I'm not entirely sure why I'd demonised biscuits as the culprit for my body size. Second, using shame as a method of accountability was super-problematic to say the least, but I had little insight into anything about that back then.

I wish I could tell you that my six years at medical school had taught me to be able to recognise and avoid fad diets, but I can't. The first thing I did to try to lose weight was drastically cut almost all the carbohydrates out of my meals . . . because carbs make you fat, right?! I wish I could have given my 24-year-old self a copy of this book after first hitting him over the head with it. I wasn't immune to believing the nutribollocks. No one is. This book isn't about making you feel bad for falling for it – it's about empowering you to make sure it doesn't happen again.

As someone with the privilege and capacity to be able to cook, I started making all my meals from scratch in order to accurately count calories. I had no real regard for nutrients; the only measurement for if I was doing well was the number on the scales.

I developed a love–hate (mainly hate) relationship with MyFitnessPal. For those of you lucky enough to have not come across it, it's a phone app where you log all your food in order to track calorie intake. Don't download it, unless you want to end up being that person who eats one chocolate from the staff room and then picks up the tray to scan the barcode with their phone. I've been there; it's not fun.

These kinds of actions impact our relationship with food, something that is incredibly important. Food is an integral part of our lives from birth until death, yet we tend to disregard the impact of disordered eating behaviours on our health. I've mentioned disordered eating a couple of times so far in this chapter without really defining what it means, so let's stop and do so now.

It's sometimes hard to be clear about things that fall under the bracket of 'unhealthy eating behaviours' and 'disordered eating'. 'Normal' eating behaviours are defined by many things: age, culture, situation and medical history, just to name a few. For example, religious fasting during Ramadan isn't automatically disordered eating, but deciding not to eat during daylight hours in the pursuit of weight loss is likely to be. Altering carbohydrate intake might be useful for a person with diabetes to manage their blood sugar levels, but what about someone without diabetes choosing not to eat them due to a fear of supposed weight gain?

Disordered eating habits are abnormal behaviours that have the potential to negatively impact your health. I think it's the difficulty of defining what is 'normal' that people really struggle with when it comes to conversations around diet. Some eating habits are disordered without question, but many are very context-dependent. *We are not meant to all eat the same.* Social media is full of false promises telling you that if you eat a certain way, you'll look a

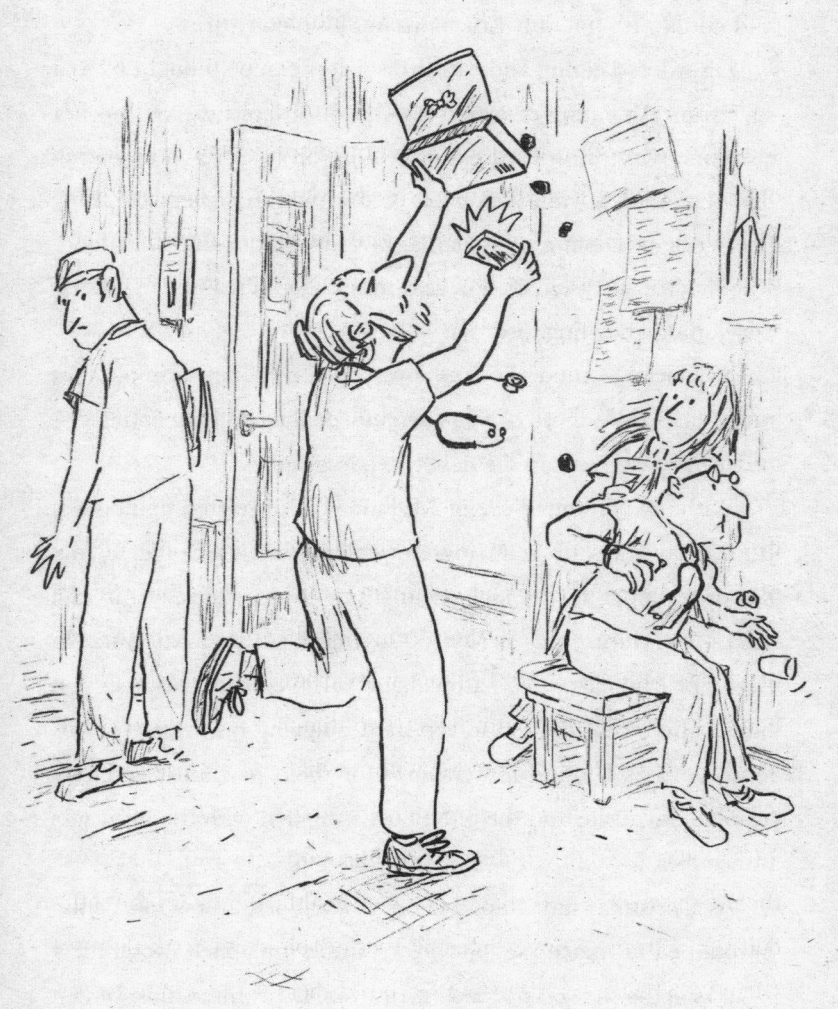

certain way, something that is complete bullshit. Our decisions around food are constantly wrapped up in our desire to be thin and not fat. It's not only ridiculous but it's bloody tiring.

Disordered eating and eating disorders can be thought of as a spectrum. All eating disorders exhibit disordered eating, but not everyone with disordered eating will go on to develop an eating disorder. Our normalisation of dieting within society certainly doesn't help. Dieting itself damages your relationship with food, whether you realise it or not, and may even increase your risk of developing an eating disorder.

Still clear as mud? Let me give you a personal example that might help (TW: those of you currently dealing with an eating disorder may want to skip the next two paragraphs).

With my continued use of MyFitnessPal, I started finding less traditional ways of reducing my calorie intake. Some of my favourite things to eat include anything with raisins, sugar and spices, but during this period of my life I cut them all out. No Eccles or fruit cakes. No oatmeal and raisin cookies. No hot cross buns. The restriction led to repeated bingeing on these types of food items as I found my cravings for them had amplified. My absolute favourite and the one that I struggled with the most was mince pies.

As Christmas time approached, I developed a new behaviour. I would eat a mince pie, but before swallowing each mouthful, I would spit the chewed-up food into the bin. In my mind, this seemed to make sense . . . yet it filled me with shame. I was always very careful to hide it, never doing it around anyone and always repositioning items in the bin so that no one else would see them.

I remember one time my housemate walked in on me as I spat into the bin, so I pretended to choke so they wouldn't suspect anything.

If what I'm talking about resonates with you, please reach out and talk to someone who can help. Don't ignore it. Either your GP or the Beat ED Charity is a great place to start (see page 256).

Who knew that ice cream could be so inflammatory?

Let's get back to my Instagram account, which I initially chose to call @unfattening. I went as far as buying customised running trainers with that word on the sides and was even considering getting it as a tattoo. Thank goodness I didn't.

A couple of years after starting the account I'd somehow managed to convince over thirty thousand people to follow me despite only posting pictures of food and the occasional transformation photo. I even had the phrase 'evidence-based fitness' in my bio. Cringe. My world revolved around weight loss and diet culture and having lost a fair bit of weight at that point I thought myself an expert; a common theme among those online from Z-list celebrities to healthcare professionals.

Unbeknownst to me, it would be a random conversation about ice cream that really started to shake things up.

Hands up who remembers when Halo Top was launched in the UK? It was sold as a 'guilt-free', high-protein, low-calorie ice cream – one where you were literally encouraged to eat the whole tub. I placed it on a pedestal and sang its praises on my Instagram, tagging the company in my stories in the hope that they would sponsor me so I didn't have to keep paying the extortionate price it was sold at. I did get some free samples at one point, probably in an attempt to stop me hassling them.

It had become commonplace for my followers to send me screenshots of content online to ask for my thoughts or for me to debunk something. In 2018 I was linked to an Instagram story by Laura Thomas (@laurathomasphd), a registered nutritionist and intuitive-eating counsellor based in London. In it she seemed to be bashing Halo Top for encouraging bingeing and asking why anyone would want to choose it over the real thing . . . or that's how I remember it anyway. I remember feeling attacked, almost personally, so much so that I felt compelled to send her the following message:

> 'Except it tastes almost IDENTICAL to regular ice
> cream and means that I can eat a decent amount without
> cramming empty calories and sugar into my body!!! I get
> that diet culture can be a bad thing, but why attack the
> premise of making a high-sugar, high-calorie product
> better for your body and your health? I don't get it.'

I really didn't. I didn't understand why a low-calorie alternative could be anything but a good thing. Laura could (and probably should) have just ignored me at this point, but she was kind enough to send the following in reply:

> 'Well I think we have to be careful about calling ice
> cream an empty calorie, it can be a source of vitamins,
> minerals and protein for people. It's really the marketing

that's problematic here; it's not even a suggestion but an expectation that people will eat the entire tub because it's "healthy". It's also a lot less satisfying so you end up eating more than a scoop or two of the regular stuff. That will leave people feeling bloated, cramping and potentially running to the loo (based on high soluble fibre). This type of product lures people into a false sense of healthy as opposed to developing a good relationship to food (which means eating a wide variety of foods without feeling guilty or "bad" for the occasional bowl of ice cream).'

I had never heard anyone speak about food in this way before. What she was saying made sense, but the mindset I was in at the time wouldn't allow me to admit that it did. It challenged things I believed about food: even the simple statement of being able to just eat a scoop or two of ice cream was something foreign to me. At that time, I was refusing to buy food items that I enjoyed but considered 'unhealthy' as I ending up bingeing on them. That internal conflict made me want to know more and led to a response that I think even surprised myself:

'I greatly respect your experience and expertise and I would honestly love to meet up and chat with you . . . I want to be medically accurate with the advice that I give out and would honestly love to pick your brain.'

Laura very graciously agreed to meet me. The following month I travelled on the train into central London and took up her entire afternoon asking question after question. I left even more conflicted, but realising that even if just a *tiny* amount of what she'd told me about weight, health and dieting was true, I needed to do some more digging. It was my first step towards the concepts of weight inclusivity and 'intuitive eating', and it was a game-changer.

Willing to be wrong

The next ten months were interesting. I read research I'd never been exposed to before, listened to hours upon hours of different podcasts and followed a whole slew of new faces on social media. I can imagine that the non-diet accounts on Instagram were probably very confused as to why someone called @unfattening was suddenly interested in their content! It's really telling looking back on my feed during that time, as I can see the conflict in my head that I was struggling to put into words. The longer it went on, the more I realised that a lot of the things I was promoting were not only full of contradictions but incredibly problematic.

After I stopped actively encouraging weight loss, I began to be challenged about the appropriateness of my Instagram username. I resisted. Like, *seriously* resisted. I liked that @unfattening felt catchy and I didn't want to let go of it. I convinced myself and anyone who would listen that the reason it was okay for me to keep using it was because it attracted the perfect kind of audience I was wanting to reach. I disregarded the harm it could cause, because in my head, the end justified the means. My ego got in the way.

In January of 2019, ironically peak 'diet' time, I finally bit the bullet and changed my social media name to @drjoshuawolrich.

This turned out to be a massive weight off my shoulders. Since then, my presence online has evolved into one challenging weight stigma, health inequity, nutribollocks and fad diets.

I'm hoping there are going to be things in this book that challenge what you believe to be true about your health and nutrition. Changing someone's opinion on a topic usually requires a level of trust not often reached through pages of text, but I'm confident that my candidness so far will have helped to build the necessary foundations. Let's get started.

2.

YOUR WEIGHT DOES NOT DEFINE YOUR HEALTH

I remember going to my mother as a teenager and asking her advice on how to lose weight. With complete conviction and in an attempt to help, she told me that all I needed to do was make sure I only ate sandwiches that had less than 10g of fat in them. I believed her without question, and it took a surprisingly long time before I was able to buy a sandwich without that advice impacting my choices.

Nutribollocks is pervasive. How many of you were told similar things by a loved one, be that friends or family? Just recently, completely unsolicited, a fellow doctor at work described to me the supposed benefits of removing all carbs for weight loss. He then went one step further and started praising the virtues of the ketogenic diet before I had to stop him as I felt my blood pressure rising.

The overwhelming majority of nutribollocks, be that online or in person, is sold with the promise of weight loss in some shape or form. In recent years, as the public have become slightly wiser to the fact that 'dieting' is neither a reliable nor risk-free endeavour, much of it has been rebranded on the promise of health. Instead of juice fasting being just for weight loss, it's now a 'cleanse' that will 'reset your metabolism'. Don't be fooled by clever marketing – it's still bollocks.

When I tell people that I'm a doctor who follows a Health at Every Size® (HAES) approach[4], most people assume that means I don't believe weight can have *any* impact on health. That's not the case. Healthcare tends to follow what's known as a 'weight-normative' approach, where a focus on weight and weight loss is used to try to define health and wellbeing. This ends up resulting in the discrimination of those who don't fit within its narrow definition. HAES, however, encourages patients to be treated with a 'weight-inclusive' approach.

This means we should be emphasising that health is *incredibly* multifaceted and that the link with weight is nowhere near as straightforward as people make it out to be. We should be publicly acknowledging and refusing to stay silent about the harmful impacts of weight stigma. We, as doctors, have to stop indiscriminately advising weight loss to our patients when we have no guarantee that it's going to improve health or be sustainable over the long term. Healthcare must be inclusive and accessible for *all* patients, regardless of their weight. This is not the case at the moment and it has to change. I will go into more detail about this later on in the chapter.

There are several things that society has conditioned us to believe about our health and body weight, and by the end of this chapter I hope to have started to make you challenge their legitimacy. Even something like the link between body weight and type 2 diabetes isn't as straightforward as people insist (we will look at that in much more depth later, in chapter 4). This will be a bit of a whistle-stop tour of what are absolutely *massive* topics, so do continue to explore them after finishing this book.

Acknowledging privilege first

I'm white, middle class and male, all of which make me incredibly privileged. Often when it's implied or stated that someone is privileged it can make them feel defensive or upset. They may have worked really hard for what they've accomplished and may have overcome many obstacles to accomplish it; the word privilege can make a person feel as though that work is being diminished. I know I used to feel that way.

Yet acknowledging our privilege doesn't automatically mean we were raised by wealthy parents, had everything handed to us or didn't have to do much other than just show up. Having privilege implies nothing about whether or not we've had a difficult life. Privilege means that some of us have advantages over others for any number of reasons we can't control – the country we're born in, the colour of our skin or our socio-economic status, to name just a few. In a nutshell: even when things haven't come easy for us, we can still have privileges that others don't have.

The reason I've chosen to talk about this so early on is because it's crucially relevant to *every single* conversation involving food and health.

I recently received a comment on my social media page that read:

'When did you change from health and nutrition
information to social justice warrior statements about
privilege?'

Health and nutrition are *inherently* socio-economic issues and ones
of privilege. I am privileged to have the time to cook. I am privileged to be able to afford fresh fruit and vegetables and own a
fridge to be able to keep food from rotting too quickly. I am privileged to have the time, physical and mental capacity to exercise.
When we wilfully ignore all of this, whether or not we engage in
health behaviours becomes a moral blame game . . . and health
should never be a moral blame game. If you only take away one
thing from this book, I'm happy for it to be that (even if you choose
to keep juicing celery).

If acknowledging my privilege makes me a social justice warrior, I'm good with it. I accept the pejorative term.

Social determinants of health

'Health inequalities and the social determinants of health
are not a footnote . . . they are the main issue.'[5]
— *Sir Michael Marmot, Professor of Epidemiology
and Public Health at University College London*

The vast majority of our health is influenced by things we have very
little control over. An ignorance of this fact causes people to look
down on others who, in their opinion, simply 'aren't choosing to

prioritise their health'. If you've ever been subject to weight stigma, you'll likely recognise this sentiment immediately. This 'personal responsibility' rhetoric couldn't be further from the truth and is *incredibly* stigmatising.

Social determinants of health are responsible for around 70 per cent of the length and quality of our lives. They refer to the circumstances that have shaped and still impact the conditions in which we live and have been grouped into five different categories by the World Health Organization (WHO):

1. Healthcare access and quality
2. Education access and quality
3. Social and community context
4. Economic stability
5. Neighbourhood and environment

All of these are hugely interconnected. For example, being born in higher economic stability will mean that you are likely to live in an area of the world with better air and water quality, have access to better hospital care and be more likely to have a higher level of education. These all mean that you will have better overall health and a higher life expectancy before we even get to health behaviours like diet and exercise that we have slightly more control over.

The belief that anyone can lift themselves out of poverty and improve their health if they try hard enough isn't one that matches with reality. It's a nice sentiment, but the truth is that in the UK and US it can take at least five generations (150 years) for the

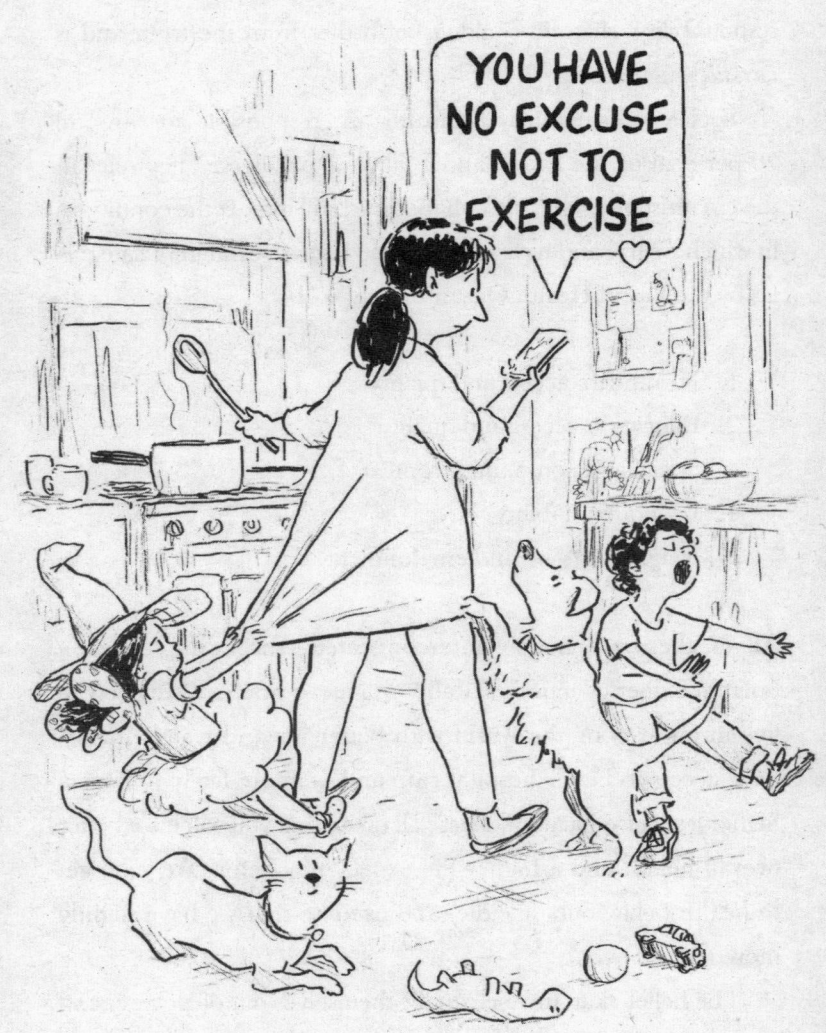

child of a poor family to get to a position where they're able to earn the average national income[6]. This is why it's so important to acknowledge the privileges we have so we can use them to advocate for those experiencing both health inequality and inequity.

Inequality refers to the uneven distribution of health resources, usually as a result of things unable to be directly changed such as genetics or lack of resources. On the other hand, health *inequity* is the unfair, avoidable differences in health as a result of things such as discrimination and politics. The latter is the biggest reason why people at a higher body weight experience poorer healthcare and poorer outcomes.

Food inequity

It's common to think of government guidelines around diet as easy to follow, but food inequity means that the poorest 10 per cent of UK households would need to spend *74 per cent* of their disposable income on food to meet Public Health England's Eatwell Guide recommendations[7]. This compares to the richest 10 per cent only having to spend 6 per cent of their disposable income. Eating a nutritious diet is a privilege that many simply cannot afford . . . yet we stigmatise by treating it as a personal responsibility.

To add to the problem, over ten million people in the UK[8], around 16 per cent of the population, live in what are known as 'food apartheids'; areas of food insecurity where poverty, poor public transport and lack of big supermarkets severely limit access to affordable fresh fruit and vegetables. Compounding the issue further, one million people in the UK are without a fridge, two million without a cooker and three million without a freezer[9]. Access to fruit and vegetables becomes irrelevant if you can't store them.

The average body weight is higher among those living in the most deprived areas of the UK (a trend that's also seen in other high-income nations[10]). Poverty, therefore, seems to play a part in influencing body size. The accusation that 'people just need to eat less to lose weight' becomes hard to justify as we start to understand the bigger picture, doesn't it?

Harmful assumptions

We live in a society with such a deep-rooted fear of being fat that we refuse to entertain the possibility that it might not define our health. We justify our position by claiming 'being slim' is about being healthy, when in fact that's often just a cover. Don't believe me? Here's a thought experiment for you: if you had to choose between being healthy and fat, or unhealthy and thin, which would it be? The fact that your brain hesitated is exactly what I'm talking about.

The assumption that weight defines our health is something we need to be questioning whenever it comes up. It's so engrained that we judge the effectiveness of any health-seeking behaviour based on whether or not it's resulted in weight loss. Take exercise as a perfect example. Regular movement is amazing for your health, but many people will only start doing it because they've been told it will make them lose weight. When this doesn't happen, disillusion sets in and activity levels fall again.

Making health all about weight is not only nonsense but it can actually lead to people disregarding behaviours that are great for them.

Let's clear up any potential confusion at the start. The extremes of body weight, at either end of the spectrum, can have a negative impact on your health. That goes for pretty much everything in life, from drinking water to how much you sleep. Having said that, it can still be very difficult to tease out whether it's *actually* body fat that's causing a problem or something else. Our health is incredibly multifaceted.

The lack of nuance around weight is propagated by the insistence of the medical community on using the body mass index (BMI) to categorise patients and determine health status. As we go forward, I will be writing the words 'ob*se' and 'ob*sity' with asterisks. These words are overwhelmingly used to discriminate and I want this book to be as inclusive as possible; I will not be a part of labelling someone with an assumed health status based on their weight (I also avoid these words in my clinical work). 'Overweight' means absolutely nothing either (over *what* weight?) but doesn't *quite* carry with it the pain of the others. My personal opinion is that these terms shouldn't be used at all, but considering what we'll be discussing, they will sometimes be helpful for clarity.

You will also find me using the word 'fat' as a descriptor in this book. This might feel weird at first as the word is still in the process of being deliberately reclaimed as the simple descriptor that it should be. Fat should not be an insult. The more we use it in normal language the less negative power it holds.

Body mass index

To understand how the medical world's reliance on the BMI came to be, we need to go back almost 200 years to a Belgian mathematician called Adolphe Quetelet. He's credited with founding the field of anthropometry (the measurement of the human body) in his pursuit to define the 'average' man. He created a calculation involving the weight and height of a group of white Western European men in order to find what he considered the 'ideal' weight.

From a statistical perspective it was designed as a way of measuring average weight at a population level, not individually (something that may feel like semantics but really isn't). How is the average weight of one ethnic group from two centuries ago meant to accurately determine the average weight of individuals of all ethnicities and genders . . . let alone their health status? Unsurprisingly it doesn't.

Quetelet's original work had nothing to do with health, but this changed during the first half of the 20th century. American life insurance companies needed to find a new way of determining how much to charge people for their coverage, so they took inspiration from Quetelet's calculation and started compiling their own data on height and weight. Despite none of this being based on any sort of scientific research, it was still used as a justification to give more expensive insurance quotes.

It didn't take long before doctors across the country also started to use these newly created insurance company categories as a convenient way to assume the health of their patients. A few decades later they reverted to using the original equation Quetelet had created after determining it was 'slightly better' for estimating body fat . . . even though research showed it was only accurate in doing that about half of the time[11]. Raise your hand if you're starting to realise just how unscientific this all is?

Now named the Body Mass Index, the measure was officially approved for use across the US in 1985[12]. The decision was made to label adults with a BMI of over 27.8 (men) or 27.3 (women) as unhealthy. Why those values? Well, they 'arbitrarily' (their word not mine) decided that a weight increase of 20 per cent higher than 'desirable' would fit the bill. Not exactly evidence-based healthcare.

A decade later, a lobbying group convinced the WHO to lower the cut-offs for both men and women to 25, labelling them as 'overweight' and adding a new category of 'ob*se' at a BMI of 30. The members of this lobbying group not only ran weight-loss clinics[13] but received the majority of their funding from the only two pharmaceutical companies that made weight-loss drugs at the time. Questionable, to say the least.

You might think this is my own bias looking for conspiracy, but even a cursory glance at the evidence used to lower the cut-offs shows otherwise. The research presented to the WHO by the lobbying group only found a relationship between increasing BMI and health above a BMI of 40[14], meaning that their own report should have *raised* the cut-offs, not lowered them. That wouldn't have benefited the growing weight-loss industry though, would it? It's not even funny how unacceptable that is.

A few years later the US followed suit and as Lindo Bacon, author of *Health at Every Size*, writes, 'one magical night in June of 1998 twenty-nine million Americans went to bed with average figures and woke up fat . . . with a presumed increased risk of type 2 diabetes, hypertension, and atherosclerosis and a government prescription for weight loss.'[4]

The BMI would never pass scientific standards if proposed today, yet because we've been using it for over half a century it's embedded in our healthcare systems and our research. Every single piece of research that looks at the relationship between BMI and health, or BMI and disease risk, carries with it the inconsistencies of a flawed measure. That doesn't mean it's all automatically useless, but it's a problem that needs to be taken into consideration . . . and rarely ever is.

Is the BMI 'good enough'?

People will try to argue away the fact that the BMI isn't perfect by claiming that it correlates with health most of the time. Does it though? For reference, the current BMI categories for both men and women are set as follows:

below 18.5	underweight
18.5–24.9	healthy weight
25.0–29.9	overweight
30 and above	ob*se (often subdivided further)

One of the biggest pieces of research we currently have on the matter of BMI and mortality comes from 2018 and uses data from

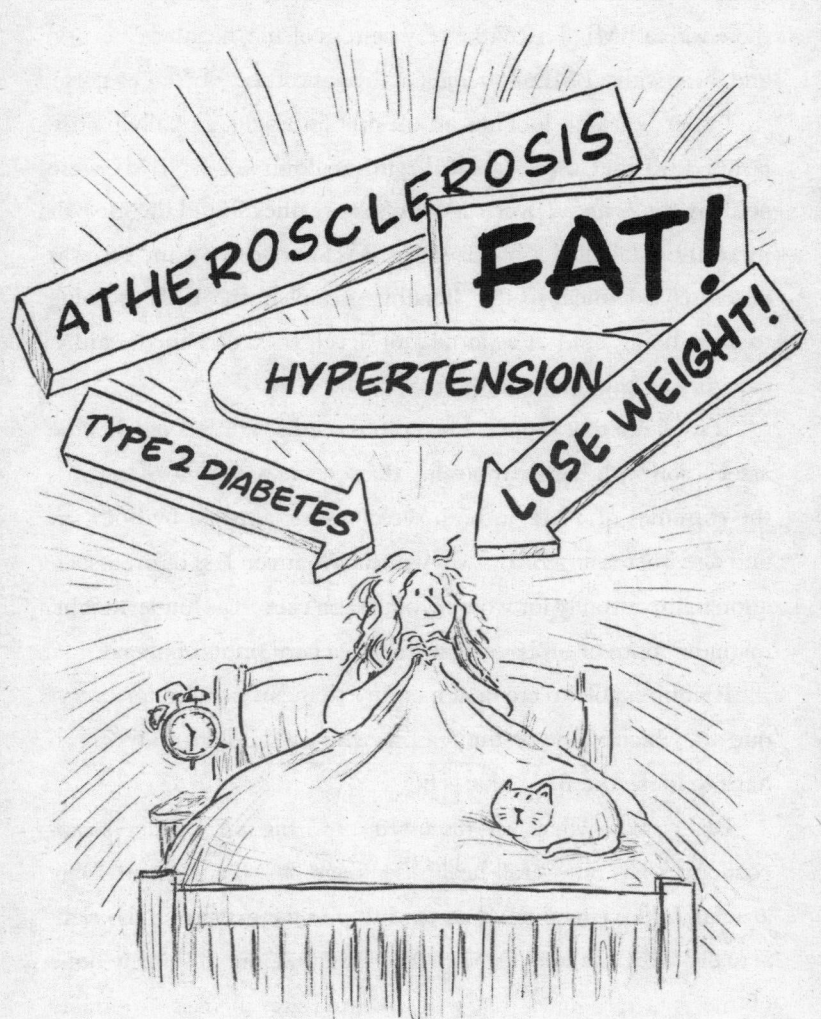

3.6 million adults in the UK[15]. It showed that the 'overweight' category is essentially useless, with no difference in mortality between those with a BMI of 18.5 (the very bottom of the 'healthy' category) and those with a BMI of 30 (right at the start of the 'ob*se' category).

Other research looking at 2.9 million adults globally[16] similarly found that those labelled with an 'overweight' BMI were actually the *healthiest* overall. What's more, they found the mortality of those labelled 'ob*se', with a BMI between 30 and 35, was absolutely identical to the 'healthy' group! If the BMI is going to keep being used at a population level, shouldn't the 'healthy' category at *least* range between 18.5 and 30?

It's still not that simple. The graphs on the right[15] show that the association with higher mortality that occurs as we move towards the extremes of BMI (in both directions) is affected by both sex and age. Increasing BMI is shown to have much less of an association with mortality for women, but being classed as 'underweight' might be more of an issue. Age follows a very similar pattern.

It's impossible to create a measure that can be used for everyone . . . which is one of the reasons why we should stop trying so hard to make the BMI charts fit.

Remember when we discussed how big an impact socio-economics has on overall health (see page 36)? Guess what? Only around 1 per cent of the data used to plot the graphs on the right actually takes this into account. Not only that, but absolutely none of the data recognises that weight stigma also increases mortality risk[17] regardless of an individual's size (we'll get to more on that in a bit). In simple terms, this is like doing research into the causes of lung cancer and not noting down if the participants smoked cigarettes.

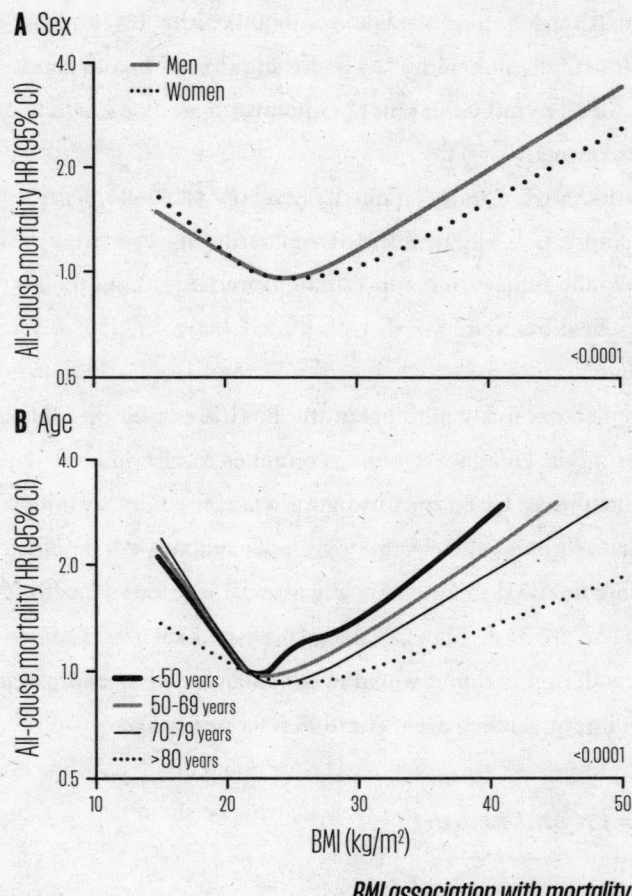

BMI association with mortality

As if it couldn't get any worse, using the BMI to plot graphs at a population level is one thing, but using it to determine the health of an individual is even *more* unreliable and simply leads to bad healthcare. When metabolic health is properly investigated by blood tests and observations including blood pressure, we find:

- Almost a third of people with a 'healthy' BMI are actually unhealthy[18]. The assumption of health can lead to individuals not being investigated or treated properly.
- A third of those labelled 'ob*se' (BMI 30–34.9) are metabolically healthy[19]. Despite this, they are universally subject to inappropriate comments about their health and told to diet.

Many doctors freely admit that the BMI is terrible, yet refuse to stop using it. Healthcare policy continues to discriminate against patients purely based on this figure when it comes to things like fertility treatment and elective joint replacements. We should never be using the BMI to automatically assume someone's health. *It has to stop.* We are more than capable of assessing current health status and encouraging things we know are guaranteed to improve matters, without needing a patient to step foot on a scale.

Body fat and health

After throwing the BMI in the bin and setting it on fire, I'd like to address the question of whether higher levels of body fat can negatively affect our health at all, as nuance is important.

The quick answer is: it depends on where in the body the fat is stored.

Aside from being a storage of energy, fat tissue is also considered an endocrine organ due to its ability to produce numerous different things such as hormones and growth factors[20]. It also has

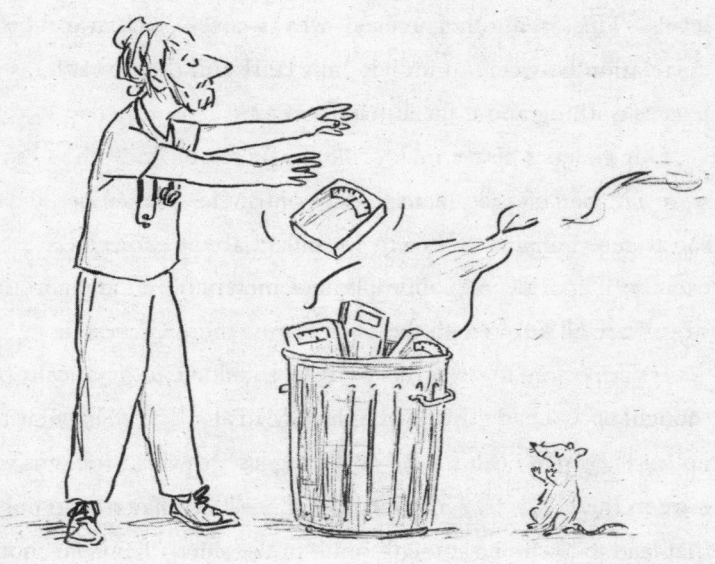

a role in regulating processes like our hunger, energy expenditure and immunity. Its function and activity changes depending on its location within the body and can have a positive or negative impact on health as a result.

The majority of our fat tissue is stored subcutaneously (just underneath the skin) with the rest being both visceral (around the organs in the abdomen) and within muscle. The strongest evidence we have suggests that increasing visceral fat has the biggest potential harmful impact on our health[21], with subcutaneous fat around the abdomen coming in second. Research has shown that increased subcutaneous fat in the hips and thighs is actually *protective* for metabolic health in adults of all ages[22], something that might be as a result of improving hormone levels. This is another reason why we see such a rubbish correlation between an individual's BMI and their health, as it tells us nothing about fat distribution.

Our genetics play a major role in where our body chooses to store fat, but lifestyle factors also contribute. Remember those social determinants of health we talked about earlier? Lack of exercise[23], poor sleep quality[24], lack of dietary fibre[25] and chronic stress[26] are all linked with the body storing more visceral fat.

It's important to stress that body fat shouldn't automatically be thought of as a bad thing; higher levels can also be associated with an *improvement* in health. One of the biggest growing problems we have in the UK is fragility fractures. Conditions like osteoporosis that lead to low bone strength result in the elderly being far more likely to break bones when they fall over. If this is a broken hip, the risk of death within a year can be up to 30 per cent[27]. Higher levels of body fat in postmenopausal women are actually *protective*[28] against both osteoporosis and the mortality associated with fragility fractures. Prior to the menopause, lower levels of fat can have negative impacts on hormone production and can lead to a condition where periods stop for several months (hypothalamic amenorrhea). This has been linked to an increased risk of cardiovascular disease and reduced bone density[29].

Body fat can also be protective when we get sick. People living with chronic diseases such as heart failure and kidney disease have a *lower* risk of death as their weight increases. Fat patients are also more likely to survive admission to an intensive care unit when severely unwell[30], something that continued to be true during the COVID-19 pandemic[31]. This fact is particularly damning when you realise that BMI can be considered a comorbidity (a pre-existing medical condition) when determining a patient's suitability for admission to ICU, despite there being no actual evidence to justify rejecting them based on their weight.

Even in situations where body fat might be having a negative impact on health, it still doesn't mean that weight loss is automatically the answer, or the only thing that will improve matters. Research has shown that healthy lifestyle habits (eating five or more vegetables and fruits daily, exercising regularly, consuming alcohol in moderation and not smoking) have the ability to positively impact health, regardless of size[32]. The 'mortality difference' in individuals starting with a 'normal' and 'ob*se' BMI completely disappeared between groups in those who followed all four habits. Other research has backed this up by showing that increasing cardiorespiratory fitness alone might have the ability to completely remove any association that higher BMI has with mortality[33].

The assumption that weight defines our health is not only untrue but incredibly disempowering. Let it go.

Weight loss is not simply a matter of willpower

How many times have you heard someone say the secret to weight loss is 'just eat less and move more'? It's a bit like telling someone that being rich is as simple as just earning more money and not spending as much. While the premise might be technically correct the reality is far more complex than the sentiment would imply.

If we consume more energy than we're using over a certain period of time, that energy ends up being stored in the body as fat. The opposite occurs when we consume less energy than we need. The complexity comes when you realise just how many factors there are that influence both the energy we consume and the amount of energy our body is using.

In 2007, a Foresight project commissioned by the UK government led to a report in which they identified over 100 different factors that influence this 'energy balance'. It confirmed what people have known for a long while – weight gain cannot be blamed on one individual thing. It would be impossible to be able to go through all 100, but here are some of the key elements to give you an idea:

- Biology: amount of muscle, distribution of body fat, childhood growth, gut efficiency, genetic predisposition, level of appetite, metabolism.
- Individual psychology: stress, level of focus on weight and size, level of focus on food control, social interaction.
- Social psychology: media consumption, cultural valuation of food, smoking, exposure to food advertising.
- Food consumption: variety, energy-density, alcohol, convenience, availability, speed of eating, portion size.
- Food environment: cost, employment, pressure to cater for different tastes.
- Individual activity: childhood activity, occupational activity, transport use, recreational activity.

- Activity environment: cost of physical exercise, safety of walking, access to physical exercise, unemployment.

That's only about a third of them. It's important to note that all of these factors are interlinked as well. Take *stress* as an example. This can impact *level of appetite* in either direction and increase the risk of *smoking*, which in turn may actually suppress the *level of appetite* while reducing the ability to undertake *recreational activity*.

Assuming someone isn't losing weight because they're just not trying hard enough is not only stigmatising but utter nonsense. It's far more complicated.

Picture yourself working two jobs; you don't have the time or energy when you come home to be able to cook a meal from scratch like social media keeps saying you should be doing and you're starting to feel shame because of it. You live in an area without a big supermarket and not owning a car means you don't have the ability to drive to one. Instead, your only option is the corner shop or the fast-food outlet within walking distance from your home. Finding something to feed you and your two children isn't easy, but you manage to make do with what little is on offer that you can afford. You live in a constant state of stress that you're not giving them food that is as healthy as you would like, but you don't have many other options. You've always had issues with insecurities around what you look like, so you decide to skip dinner for a week in order to lose some weight. It works, but you can't avoid dinner forever as you start to struggle with lack of energy at work. Not only has your relationship with food taken another hit, but the weight comes back again like it always does.

I'm privileged enough not to have experienced anything quite like this, but for several million people in the UK this is not far from reality. The overwhelming number of people who have lost weight and are now trying to sell you their 'success' story have no insight into any of this either. Each of us will be experiencing a number of different factors that can affect our weight in either direction – from having a child to working night shifts or simply the stress of living through a global pandemic.

Weight regain is almost inevitable

You might have heard of the old adage that 95 per cent of diets fail, but is that completely true? The reality isn't much better. The best research we have at the moment looked at 27 weight-loss studies that followed their participants for five years after their chosen diet[34]. More than 80 per cent of the weight was regained by the end of the five-year period, with more than half of it having already been gained back after just two years. Every single weight-loss study showed that participants regain weight before the end of the follow-up period.

People will often point to the National Weight Control Registry in the US (set up to investigate the characteristics of long-term weight loss) as proof that weight loss can be successful[35]. There are a couple of things to mention here. First, this is a self-selected registry, meaning that people who have lost weight *choose* to register. As such, any statistics of long-term weight loss are going to be overestimated as people who regained weight aren't likely to join. Second, the description given of people who are counted as successes isn't very encouraging: they engage in high levels of physical activity, eat a low-calorie diet and don't deviate across weekdays or weekends. More than half of them report that they are still actively trying to lose weight, with similar numbers weighing themselves at least once a day. I'm not sure what measure of success you would use, but to me, that's not it.

Hardwired to resist weight loss

Resisting weight loss has been beneficial from an evolutionary perspective for millennia. For most of human existence, food was a scarcity, so any energy we managed to consume was held onto as much as possible. The Western world is now very much in a state of plenty in comparison, but our biology hasn't had time to change yet.

We have an inbuilt weight-regulation system that tries to point us towards what's known as our 'setpoint', the weight that our body is most comfortable at when we're not trying to manipulate it. Metabolic ward studies (where participants are admitted to a research unit for the duration of the trial) have shown that our metabolism quickly changes to compensate for any weight change in order to bring it back to its setpoint[36].

The problem is that, with so many of us ignoring our hunger and fullness cues while deliberately trying to manipulate our weight, we seem to have messed with this system. Let me give you an example:

Leptin is a hormone predominantly made in our fat cells; its presence plays a part in regulating food intake by reducing our appetite. Dieting and weight loss quickly drop levels of leptin, leaving us feeling hungry in an attempt by the body to resist what's going on. Research has suggested these low leptin levels may even increase the response of our taste buds to sugar as a way of encouraging us to specifically eat high-energy food[37] and regain the weight faster. After the dieting stops and the weight is regained, leptin levels come back up again. The issue is that a history of dieting and weight cycling (the repeated loss and regain of weight) appears to stop leptin levels returning to normal[38], leaving someone permanently hungrier and more likely to regain more weight than they lost.

If we gain weight above our setpoint, leptin usually increases to try to bring our weight back down, but after a while we can become resistant to it[39]. There is far more complexity here than I can do justice to, but the crux of the matter is that leptin is just one of the reasons why it's much easier for our setpoint to shift up rather than down. With dieting shown to be a positive predictor of weight gain[40], maybe it's time to stop dieting and accept our body for what it is.

Weight loss has never simply been a matter of willpower. Treating it as such turns our body weight into a personal responsibility, which in turn leads to overt discrimination. This brings us onto the next point.

The negative impacts of weight stigma

'Weight stigma' is discrimination or stereotyping based on a person's weight. It's far more prevalent than anyone is willing to admit. How often have you seen a TV show where the fat characters weren't portrayed as clumsy, lazy or the comedy character?

When did you last see one as the main love interest? Research has suggested that weight stigma prevalence is close to reported rates of race discrimination[41], yet it's continued to not only be socially acceptable but often encouraged by the media and government. Our culture tends to view higher body weight as being representative of a lack of moral character, bad hygiene and low levels of intelligence, just to name a few. It should go without saying that absolutely none of these are true.

This discrimination is shockingly prevalent in healthcare. Doctors have been shown to hold high levels of explicit and implicit 'anti-fat' bias[42], viewing fat patients as awkward and non-compliant. One study found that over half of patients labelled as overweight or ob*se reported receiving inappropriate comments about weight from their doctors[43].

This results in doctors denying fat patients appropriate medical care. A prime example of this is in the context of pelvic examinations for screening of conditions such as endometrial and ovarian cancer. Doctors have been shown to be more reluctant to perform these examinations when the patient is fat[44]. Are you as angry as I am yet?

Weight stigma kills. One recent example is of an anonymous patient who had gone for a cervical smear appointment[45]. The nurse who was performing the procedure complained about how the patient's fat was making her job more difficult and told her she should lose weight before coming back. The patient never returned and ended up dying at the age of 32 with metastatic cervical cancer.

This is a painful example of the reality that weight stigma in healthcare causes; patients are not only more likely to avoid appointments, but stop seeking future medical care altogether[46]. Ignorance is no longer an excuse; this stuff is *our* responsibility as healthcare professionals to fix.

Remember when I talked about internalising the weight stigma I'd experienced that led me to believe I couldn't be a good doctor if I was fat? There's research to show I'm not the only one. One study showed that when medical students internalise their experiences of weight stigma they are more likely to report both depression symptoms and substance abuse[47].

The experience of weight stigma is incredibly harmful and has been linked with numerous effects on an individual's mental and physical health[48]. This includes:

- depression, anxiety, eating disorders, suicidal thoughts and behaviours[49]
- increased blood pressure[50]
- chronic stress and inflammation[51]
- heart disease risk[52]

Put all that together and you end up with the fact that weight stigma itself has been shown to increase risk of death by nearly 60 per cent[17].

One justification I hear for why stigmatising someone for their weight is valid is that the person will lose weight. 'Tough love', if you will. This is complete and utter bullshit. Putting aside the fact that *even if it did* there is never an excuse for discrimination, weight stigma can actually promote weight gain[53]. The stress from experiencing stigma can lead to the use of food as a coping mechanism and eating more[54] while also avoiding exercise[55].

We must all start taking this seriously. Now.

The risks of intentional weight loss

It's far too common for dieting to be incorrectly seen as a risk-free endeavour; one of the reasons why weight loss is advised so indiscriminately by doctors. Please know that I'm not here to chastise you for wanting to lose weight, but I am here to give you as much info as possible so that you understand the risks of attempting to do so.

We need to talk about the link between dieting and eating disorders. I'm wary here of being too dogmatic, seeing as there are many complicated reasons as to why and how people develop eating disorders, but there are some strong associations that cannot be ignored. Research has consistently shown dieting to be a risk factor for the development of all eating disorders[56], with several studies reporting that the progression from 'normal dieting' to developing an eating disorder after two years might even be as high as 10 per cent[57]. With anorexia nervosa specifically having the highest mortality rate of all mental illness[58] and one of the criteria for its diagnosis being persistent restricted food intake, it's crucial that we start paying more attention to the potential for real harm.

Diet culture takes eating disorder behaviours and normalises them. It justifies their existence by convincing you it's actually about 'improving your health'. Missing meals, counting calories, ignoring our hunger cues, drinking lots of water before eating a meal . . . all of these tactics and more are straight out of an imaginary eating disorder handbook, yet they're being promoted left, right and centre.

When weight loss is sold to us as inherently healthy, the act of going on a water fast suddenly becomes completely justifiable. We ignore all the potential negative consequences of our actions, because if we end up losing weight, all is fine.

We should not be living this way. It's illogical and it's harming our health.

For the majority of people who are fortunate not to develop an explicit eating disorder as a result of their dieting, there is still the risk of anxiety, poor self-esteem, obsession over food, the use of appetite suppressants and many other issues. Combining all of these risks with the fact that weight loss is neither guaranteed to improve health nor be sustainable over the long-term, isn't it time that we stopped pursuing weight loss? It might take a leap of faith but I promise you'll have far more success with your health when you do. Give it a go.

As I mentioned at the beginning of this chapter, these are absolutely massive topics. There's a lot here that you can read more about in your own time, and that's something I'd really encourage you to do. As we move on, you'll notice that an awful lot of the nutribollocks I'm going to address uses incorrect assumptions about weight to try to draw you in. The good news is that you're now one step ahead already.

3.

FOOD ISN'T MEDICINE

The teaching I got on nutrition/dietetics at medical school was almost non-existent. At first glance, that may seem like a failing by those in charge due to the role that nutrition plays in our overall health. It could be argued that having the ability to encourage patients in the direction of health-promoting behaviours such as diet (as opposed to only treating the patient when things go wrong) is a skill that some divisions of conventional medicine are lacking. However, seeing as I used the phrase 'at first glance' you've probably figured I'm not convinced it's that clear cut.

As doctors we treat patients as a part of a multidisciplinary team. Healthcare professionals with different areas of expertise work together to form appropriate care plans. Medical school never taught me how to design a rehab exercise programme for patients after having a hip replacement, but fortunately the physiotherapists are really good at doing that. I was never taught how to properly assess a patient's swallow after a stroke to see if they're safe to drink normal liquids without choking, but there are speech and language therapists who are trained to. Guess who else is a crucial part of the multidisciplinary team? Dietitians and nutritionists. As doctors we need to have enough knowledge to call upon the available expertise appropriately, but not so much that we end up believing we don't need help. The latter leads to poor medical care.

Now, that doesn't mean I believe diet is unimportant. Quite the opposite, which is one of the reasons why I've chosen to do a nutrition MSc. That would be a complete waste of time and money if I thought that nutrition didn't matter. I think that medical students *should* have some teaching on nutrition during medical school, but I have real concern about who would be put in charge of the curriculum. When it comes to the conversations about nutrition online, the loudest voices seem to have become medical doctors. Let me explain why I think that's a problem.

When I became interested in learning more about nutrition, I believed that reading and analysing all the papers that I was coming across wasn't a problem because I was a doctor, and being a doctor meant I 'understood science'. The issue is that medical school never taught me the following crucial fact: biomedical science is not the same as nutritional science. It's a very different skill and something I had no appreciation of.

Medical students need to be taught about nutrition by someone who understands this difference, otherwise we'll risk ending up with a whole generation of future doctors believing that food is medicine – a phrase that carries huge potential for harm, especially when used by a profession with so much authority bias. This can often be an inflammatory topic to broach, so let me clarify by saying that the majority of people who promote this rhetoric are very well meaning, but that doesn't change the fact it needs challenging. Things with potential for harm don't get a pass just because they're well-intentioned.

Nutrients are not drugs

'Hi Josh, I just wanted to share why I agree that "food is medicine" is such an important rhetoric to challenge from my own personal experience. I developed severe skin issues in my adulthood. It's been a long journey to get a diagnosis with countless hospital trips (including a three-day hospital stay once due to secondary sepsis), endless medicines and topical treatments, desperation and discomfort. I am now incredibly grateful to say my condition is under control and my skin looks and feels better than it has done in three years. This is because I'm using methotrexate injections. Without it, only steroids could keep my symptoms under control. What made that journey 1000000x harder was when people told me, or I read on the internet (it's prolific) that to cure my skin problems all I needed to do was go on a dairy-free diet, or cut out gluten, or eat tons of turmeric. Coupled with people telling me that I just needed to "stop scratching" it created a really toxic narrative that the cure lay within myself; it was up to me. If I fixed my diet, lifestyle and stopped scratching I would be healed. When I tried these things and they inevitably failed, I felt like I failed myself . . . as if I was inflicting the sleepless nights and disfigured skin on myself. It wasn't a change of diet I needed; it was methotrexate (in my case). I understand people who say food is medicine are often coming from a good place and I know it can be pursued in conjunction with conventional medicine, but I think it can also serve as a harmful distraction to people finding the medical treatment that they need and deserve.'

It's all too common for people to assume that the vitamins and minerals in food act like drugs. Take vitamin C as an example. When someone doesn't get enough it can lead to a condition called scurvy, which causes spontaneous bleeding, limb pain and ulceration of the gums and loss of teeth. When someone with scurvy consumes food that contains vitamin C the vast majority of these symptoms resolve. Is this not medicine?

The way that nutrients act in the body is defined by something known as Bertrand's rule[59] (see diagram opposite).

Like the scurvy example, without enough of a certain nutrient we develop signs and symptoms that are usually pretty obvious, especially with vitamins; this is known as *deficiency*. Then come a biological range of *adequacy*, during which our body has enough of that nutrient and there is no benefit to consuming any more. Your body only needs so much; anything extra can't be used and is got rid of. With some nutrients, too much can even be harmful.

Drugs, on the other hand, are able to do things to the human body that nothing else can. They change physiology by acting outside of biological range; for example, if you continue to take

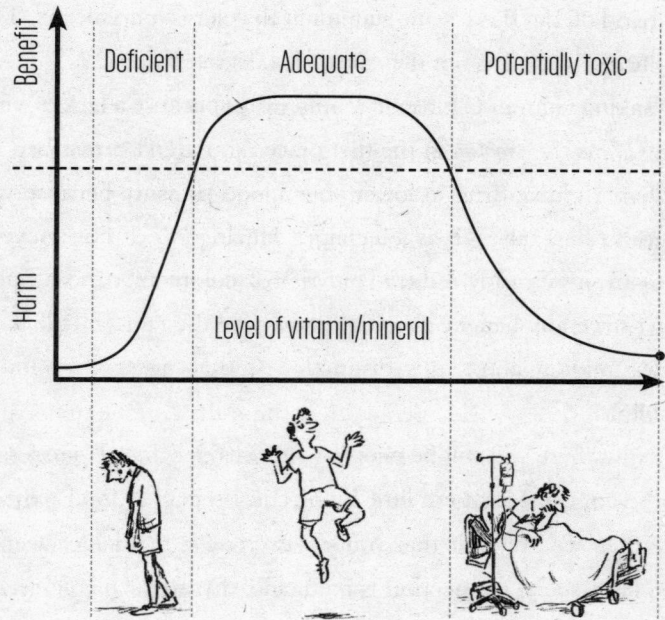

Bertrand's rule

medication for your blood pressure, it will continue to drop until you pass out. Your body can't recognise it's had enough (and get rid of it or choose to store the drug for later) like it can with the nutrients from food. Nutrients and drugs are *not* the same and it's important to acknowledge that distinction.

Is it just semantics though? After all, the dictionary definition of medicine is: 'the science and art dealing with the maintenance of health and the prevention, alleviation or cure of disease.'

We know that food *can* be preventative, just like medicine, and although having the perfect quantity of nutrients doesn't guarantee you won't get unwell, neither does medicine. So, when vitamin C is given to treat scurvy, isn't it acting like medicine?

Kind of, but there's one statement that sums it up nicely: 'The absence of a drug is not the cause of a disease'[60].

Taking vitamin C for scurvy only works because a lack of vitamin C was the *problem* in the first place. You aren't prescribed an antihypertensive drug to lower your blood pressure because you forgot to start taking it as a teenager. Having lots of fibre in your diet can significantly reduce your risk of colorectal cancer, but it won't have any benefit if you already have the cancer. A lack of understanding about this distinction is the cause of so many problems.

Now, there will still be people who consider that semantics. If that's you, can I ask for a little bit of consistency? If food is medicine then it's only fair that you say exercise is medicine, sleep is medicine, social connection is medicine, therapy is medicine . . . and you need to promote all those just as loudly. Despite the exact same logic, no one really uses those phrases because they're simply not as exciting. It's also not as easy to *sell* any of those as it is to sell a way of eating that promises to cure all of your health problems. Call me cynical if you'd like but it's the harsh reality.

Taking it to the extreme

There tend to be two different camps of people who say that 'food is medicine'. The first is usually quite moderate, such as someone with an inflammatory condition who, after seeing someone promoting oily fish for its 'anti-inflammatory' properties, now believes that fish can be medicine. The other camp is a lot more extreme, claiming that nutrition is the only thing that's needed for perfect

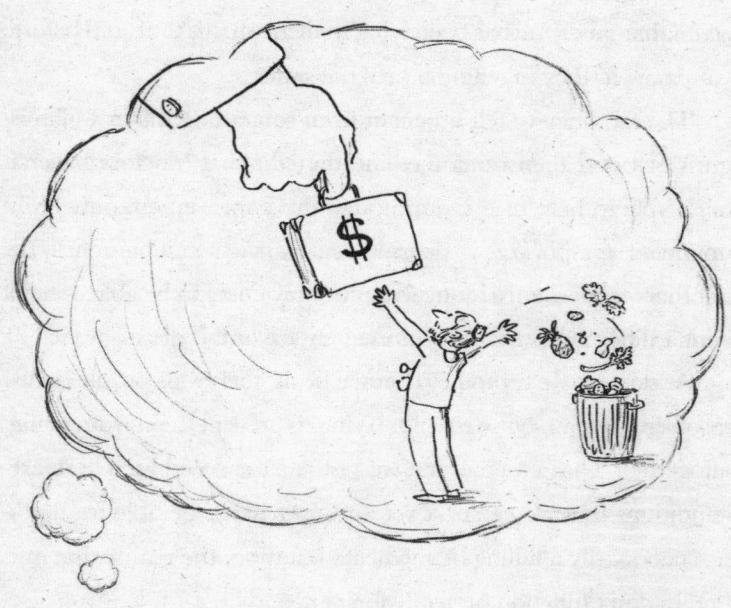

health and believes that us doctors are withholding this information because we're all paid off by Big Pharma (we're not). I doubt that any of you who have bought this book sit on that side of the fence, but if so, that would be awesome. You are exactly the kind of person I want to talk to. Please keep reading.

I think that there is a really blurred line between the two approaches, and one can so often lead into the other. Once the person with an inflammatory condition is told that by filling their diet with 'anti-inflammatory' foods they'll be able to fix their condition, it isn't long before they find others who can vouch for the claim. They then try it, feel a little better (due to a whole host of other reasons) and start wondering why their doctor didn't tell them any of this. It's at that point they start listening to those who claim that medicine has been lying to them all this time and before you know it, they're telling others the same.

The fact they've felt a benefit from something that a wellness guru has said then reinforces the thought that 'doctors haven't been able to help me.' Even though the improvement only ends up being temporary, it doesn't usually matter. There will be another wellness guru along soon who promises to be able to help with a different spurious recommendation or fad diet.

As doctors we try to help people be as healthy as possible during their lifespan, but we're not trying to prevent them from dying altogether. That's a goal that we just can't succeed at. There are conditions that we can't fix yet and may never be able to; that's not necessarily a failing of medicine but more the reality that our bodies don't function perfectly forever.

Unfortunately, the alternative promises from our growing culture of wellness can lead people further and further away from trusting their doctor. If they choose to tell their doctor about how they've recently started drinking celery juice to cure their eczema they'll often just get concern back and are even sometimes made to feel stupid . . . so they stop telling their doctor what they're doing.

Doctors have some responsibility here

So why are people looking beyond their doctors for advice? Into the gap that conventional medicine leaves open arrive disproven practices like naturopathy and 'functional' medicine. Practitioners charge hundreds for a consultation that usually just includes pseudoscientific food intolerance tests that always come back positive for gluten and dairy. Funny that.

A lot of the conditions that doctors don't currently have a lot of good answers for seem to disproportionately, or exclusively, affect women. Conservative estimates suggest that around 78 per cent of the people affected with autoimmune diseases are women[61] and into this space the wellness gurus have stepped up to sell answers.

As medical doctors we need to start accepting some responsibility for this. Bias against women from healthcare professionals has a sordid history. 'Female hysteria', for example, used to be a common medical diagnosis up until the early 20th century[62]. It was defined by a collection of vague symptoms: anxiety, nervousness, fullness in the lower abdomen, erotic fantasies, paralytic states and fainting . . . all believed to be as a result of the uterus 'choking' the patient due to sexual deprivation. Doctors even used to treat this through the entirely unacceptable practice of genital massage. This was only 100 years ago, people.

Although nothing this blatant happens today, all we have to do is look at the differences in pain management to see that we still have a lot of work to do. Women make up more of the diagnoses related to chronic pain, for example, yet the majority of the research has only been performed on men (and male mice . . .). This bias not only leads to women being left waiting longer in A&E before their pain is acknowledged[63], but when it is they're more likely than men to be given inappropriate sedatives rather than painkillers[64]. The medical community still doesn't take women's symptoms seriously, but the pseudoscientific community does. It's time to step up.

We eat food, not nutrients

By focusing on an individual nutrient, rather than the food it came from, we fall into the trap of 'reductionist nutrition'. This is an assumption that once we know the nutrients that are in a food, that food must now do all the things that the nutrients do; this leads to things like 'fish cures autoimmune disease because it contains anti-inflammatory nutrients'. This doesn't hold up for many reasons[65], but the main one is the fact that our diet simply doesn't work this way – we eat food, not nutrients. Now that doesn't mean we shouldn't be aiming to get as many nutrients as possible (this is why we generally encourage the consumption of unprocessed whole foods) but guiding this with a reductionist approach doesn't actually serve our health.

Nutrients tend to interact with each other in the context of the wider diet and lifestyle in ways that lab research just can't account for. It's very common for doctors to be the culprits of thinking about nutrition this way, as this is how drugs work! The problem is, as we've covered, nutrients aren't drugs, and the overwhelming majority of people who have studied nutrition and dietetics don't treat them as such.

If I told you that Monster energy drinks have what's known as inositol in them, a nutrient that we know has real efficacy in regards to improving symptoms for women with PCOS[66], would you believe me if I tried to sell you Monster as a cure for PCOS? Although I would imagine that most would think this sounds utterly ridiculous, people are more than happy to believe that a recipe with fish might be a cure for an inflammatory disease. Be careful not to accept 'reductionist nutrition' just because someone is proclaiming a 'natural' sounding version. It's still nutribollocks.

First do no harm

As doctors we have to make choices on a daily basis in regards to risk and benefit. Every single thing that we do in medicine has the potential for harm, even the simplest thing, like taking a blood test. When we find a better way of doing something that has the same benefit, but with less harm, we choose that route every single time. We stop using the old way because the unnecessary risk is no longer justified. Can you see where I'm going with this yet?

The use of the phrase 'food is medicine' has a lot of potential for harm. The good news is that we don't need to use it in order to express just how important food can be for our health. We shouldn't just be *hoping* that the potential to mislead people into replacing medicine with food doesn't happen – we should be *making sure* it doesn't.

One of the most worrying examples of harm is in the context of cancer treatment. Not everybody who believes that food is medicine is going to ignore conventional therapy and instead juice-fast in a cancer ranch, but everybody who goes to a cancer ranch believes that food is medicine. People die because of it. We need to acknowledge that reality and decide whether we're okay with the risk of encouraging it.

We have a saying in medicine that 'people have the right to make objectively bad decisions'. As a doctor, my job is to assess their capacity to be able to make them without projecting my morals on the situation. If someone has been convinced by a wellness guru online that juicing will cure their cancer, do they really have a full understanding of the benefits and risks when their doctor is explaining chemotherapy options to them? Is it possible to truly weigh up the available information and reject conventional treatment while believing a complete and utter lie? I'm not sure I have an answer to that.

You might have come across stories of people who claim to have proof of curing their own cancer with food . . . what's with that? Well, at risk of getting myself in trouble, they usually tend to be people who didn't have cancer in the first place. The vast majority of these stories revolve around thyroid lumps. More than 95 per cent of all thyroid nodules aren't cancerous and some of them even have the ability to go away on their own, making for the perfect, misleading, 'food cured my cancer' story. This situation is fuelled by the growing number of professionals who use their non-medical 'doctor' title to advise on people's health, despite never having set foot through the doors of a medical school. This leads to people believing they've been given an expert opinion, when in reality they've been falsely diagnosed without even having a biopsy. It's scarily dangerous.

Let's talk about cardiovascular health, as another example. It's becoming more common to see people, including some doctors, demonise medications like statins in favour of diet changes. If food is medicine then we don't need drugs, do we? The harsh reality is this: if you have elevated LDL cholesterol (a marker of cardiovascular disease) and a family history of heart disease, you can follow all of the dietary interventions we know and you would still only reduce your LDL by about 20 per cent in comparison to drug therapy[67].

Can food be used alongside medicine? 100 per cent. Should we be encouraging the dietary interventions where possible? Of course! Might they be important when someone can't tolerate medication due to side effects? I'd say so. Are they equivalent to medicine? Absolutely not.

Are you someone who uses the phrase 'food is medicine' with your patients, with your clients, or maybe just with family and friends? Please reconsider doing so. When our rhetoric has potential for harm, we need to get over ourselves and stop using it. There are much better ways of describing how important food is.

Food is food.

Medicine is medicine.

Let's stop confusing the two.

4.

STOP DEMONISING CARBS

*'In order for me to meet my goals
I'm limiting myself to no bread, no
carbs, no sugar . . .'*

BEYONCÉ

It's hard to name a popular celebrity who *hasn't* gone on a restrictive diet and told their fans about it. What makes the Beyoncé quote particularly noteworthy is the fact that whoever happened to be in charge of editing her *Homecoming* documentary decided to overlay a clip of her eating an apple as she said it.

I like to think that this person did it deliberately in order to show just how ridiculous the whole thing is, but unfortunately this kind of confusion is all too commonplace. If you were actually going to follow a no-carb diet, all fruit would officially be off the table. Also, all carbs are made from sugar, so saying 'no carbs, no sugar' is just as pointless as saying 'no meat, no chicken'.

My hope is that by the end of this chapter you will a) no longer be freaked out by the fact I just said 'all carbs are made from sugar' and b) know that removing all carbohydrates from your diet is not only a fruitless act (pun most definitely intended) but potentially damaging to both your relationship with food and your health. Please don't do it.

Our long history of demonising carbs

The promotion of a low-carb diet seems to date back to 1864 to an upper-middle-class English funeral director to the Victorian Royal Family by the name of William Banting. He lost weight after being prescribed by his ear surgeon what was essentially a low-carb diet; it's clearly not just modern doctors straying out of their lane now is it? As is very common for people after weight loss (myself included) he felt it was his duty to share what he thought of as new-found knowledge and wrote a booklet for the public recommending the diet[68]. When we look at what he wrote it's clear that diet culture and weight stigma have been alive and well for many, many years:

> 'Of all the parasites that affect humanity I do not know
> of, nor can I imagine, any more distressing than that
> of Obesity . . . [public] remarks and sneers, frequently
> painful in society, and which, even on the strongest mind,
> have an unhappy tendency.'

Hearing the honesty in Banting's words hit me pretty hard the first time I read them. This was a man so impacted by the way he'd been stigmatised for his size that, despite living in London through three smallpox epidemics, he still considered being fat the most distressing thing on earth. We haven't made much progress in 150 years, have we?

He describes the diet he was put on by his doctor as a replacement of his usual bread, butter, meat, beer, pastry and potatoes with lean meat, fish, green vegetables, fruit and wine. He was told categorically not to eat any potatoes or sugar. He reports both feeling and sleeping better within a couple of days of the dietary change, which I'm not overly surprised about to be honest!

Frustratingly, instead of realising that these benefits were undoubtedly from the introduction of nutrients into his diet in the form of vegetables (something severely lacking previously) he believed it was all down to the removal of starchy and sugary carbs. Was his previous diet based too much on the latter? Sure, but an unbalanced diet based too much on *any* one food group is never going to leave you feeling great.

Now, it's not usually advisable to diagnose someone without having met them, but I'm willing to make an exception this one time. I believe that there's a strong argument to be made that Banting had undiagnosed type 2 diabetes. He reports having struggled with his eyesight and hearing for some time, experiencing odd heart rhythms and having multiple skin abscesses. All of these signs and symptoms would make me highly suspicious of uncontrolled type 2 diabetes. The fact Banting reports that these all drastically improved after his dietary change adds even more weight to the diagnosis.

For someone with type 2 diabetes, a diet based heavily around starchy and sugary carbs has the potential to make blood glucose control difficult. Increasing fibre in the form of green veg and fruit and getting better sleep (as well as the probable reduction in visceral fat) would have greatly improved his blood glucose levels and with it the symptoms he was describing.

Banting's story isn't one proving that 'carbs make you fat'. At most it's an incredibly early example of how lifestyle changes can help in the management of type 2 diabetes. Otherwise, it's simply a story reminding us that we don't do well eating too much of one thing, especially without vegetables!

In order to be able to address the nutribollocks that revolves around carbs I'm going to give you a bit of science as to what they actually are and how our body processes them.

Carbs are made from sugar

Carbohydrates, protein and fat are the big components making up the food we eat. Together these are known as macronutrients. You may have also heard of micronutrients; this is the term given to the vitamins and minerals that don't provide energy but are needed for the proper functioning of our body, albeit in much smaller quantities.

It's important to note that with carbohydrates being one of the main building blocks of our food it's really damn hard to eat a meal that doesn't contain them in some shape or form. Carbs have been part of the human diet for over 170,000 years[69] and are ubiquitous in every culture across the globe . . . something that should make you start to question the logic of 'cutting them out' and whether it's really in the pursuit of health after all.

Spoiler alert: it's not.

The BBC has a habit of airing dodgy nutrition programmes, but *The Truth About . . . Carbs* definitely upped the bar. In one segment subsequently uploaded to YouTube with the title, 'The shocking amount of sugar hiding in your food', they asked members of the public to estimate how many sugar cubes were in different sources of carbohydrates[70].

When it came to guessing the difference between a portion of white rice and a bowl of strawberries, one participant went with five and six sugar cubes respectively. As the show dramatically revealed that the rice was actually '20 sugar cube equivalents', the camera panned back to the guesser, who simply stated: 'I'm not eating rice no more'.

Is it acceptable to mislead the population with fear-mongering demonstrations and mess with their relationship with food? Of course it isn't. I'm already tired of the nonsense being spread by low-carb zealots on social media, but seeing it on one of the most trusted TV channels in the UK really angered me.

Now you may be reading this and thinking, 'Hold up Josh, you said back at the beginning of the chapter that "all carbs are made from sugar", so why is this misleading?' The answer to this question will become clear as we go on, but for now remember that just as facts about weight can be used to stigmatise, facts about carbs can be used to fear-monger and mislead.

Classifying carbohydrates

We tend to categorise carbohydrates under the labels of: sugars, starch and dietary fibre. Let's look at them each in turn.

Sugars

Sugars are the generic name for any sweet-tasting simple carbohydrates, not just the stuff that some British people insist on stirring into their tea.

Sugars act as the building blocks by which all carbohydrates are made. There are several different types, but the main two to know are glucose and fructose. They are made by plants, not only to be used as an energy source so that they can grow but packed into fruit to encourage other species like our own to eat them and help spread their seeds.

The only real exception to sugars being found in plants is lactose, found in animal milk. Sugars really aren't scary. Is an apple scary? Sugars are simply energy for us to be able to function and live on.

Starch

In the same way that we as humans mainly store energy in the form of fat, plants store energy in the form of starch (complex carbohydrates). These are long chains of up to two million glucose units that by this point don't taste sweet anymore. This group is all about vegetables: cruciferous veg such as cauliflower, broccoli and cabbage; root veg including potatoes; legumes such as peas, beans and lentils; and grains including rice, oats and wheat. Anything made from flour, from bread to pasta, also counts. The vast majority of these require cooking before consumption as the heat starts breaking down the long chains of glucose and makes them easier to digest; you'd find it pretty hard to eat a raw potato!

Complex carbohydrates are where we tend to get the most micronutrients (vitamins and minerals) and also where we get our fibre.

Dietary fibre

Dietary fibre is the term used to encompass all the other carbohydrates in plants that we can't digest properly. Some types of fibre are able to be fermented by the bacteria in our gut to keep the cells of our colon healthy and reduce our risk of colon cancer[71]. The rest helps to prevent us from getting constipated by forming the bulk of our stool.

Sweetcorn is a good visual example to explain this. Each kernel has an outer layer that is mainly fibre and a mixture of complex and simple carbohydrates inside. If you don't chew it properly the fibre prevents it from being digested by your gut and you see them come out intact at the other end!

The vast majority of us don't eat anywhere near enough fibre[72]. Not only does it lower levels of cholesterol and cardiovascular risk, it reduces your risk of colon cancer and type 2 diabetes[73]. In a nutshell, eat more fibre. It's stupidly good for you.

Bonus: Refined carbohydrates

This term gets used quite a bit. It's another way to describe sugars, but the word also gets used to denote something that's been processed. Take white flour; it's mainly starch and hence a complex carbohydrate, but the processing that ends up removing most of the fibre also earns it the label 'refined'.

Carbohydrate digestion

One of the reasons why a lot of the nutribollocks around carbs continues to spread is because many of us don't really understand how our bodies digest and absorb them. It's why the bowl of rice = 20 sugar cubes analogy doesn't help us.

Let's start off with an indisputable fact: *the simple sugar glucose is the main preferred source of energy for our body*. After we've eaten carbs the most important job for our gut is to break everything down into simple sugars so that they're small enough to be absorbed into our blood stream. This then causes a rise in what's known as our blood glucose levels (a.k.a. blood sugar levels). Certain things can slow down this process, such as fibre, allowing for a more gradual rise.

You'll have probably been told that a 'spike' in blood glucose levels is automatically bad for you and should always be avoided. First, research has shown that only about 4 per cent of healthy individuals have what would be classed as 'spikes'[74] after a high-sugar meal. Second, there's no current evidence that this will actually lead to problems down the line, despite the myth that eating sugar gives you diabetes (we'll cover that later in this chapter). Slowing down the absorption of sugars from our gut is a good thing when it comes to having longer-term energy after eating, but you don't need to be afraid if that's not always the case.

Your brain is specifically dependent on sugar as its main source of energy. Did you know that over an average day the brain uses about 20 per cent of the body's total supply[75]? That's why people often end up feeling so crap when depriving them- selves with a low-carb diet! Knowing this, it makes sense that our bodies are designed to use glucose from the blood as efficiently as possible.

The main hormone responsible for this is insulin. As levels of glucose rise in our blood after digesting and absorbing the carbo- hydrates from a meal, insulin gets released from our pancreas, which then goes to work. It enables our cells to take the glucose from the blood so it can then be used for energy.

Now, we tend to have a bigger rise in blood glucose levels after a meal than is needed all in one go, so insulin also helps to manage this surplus for later. It stimulates the liver to not only store some of it in long chains as glycogen, but also convert it into body fat. All this means that between meals, when our blood glucose levels would otherwise fall too low, there are stores of glucose ready to be put back into the blood rather than us having to eat every couple of hours. We'd never be able to sleep otherwise! Insulin is one of the most important hormones in the body.

When the latest wellness guru is trying to convince you that a low-carb diet is the cure-all for health they'll often justify it by

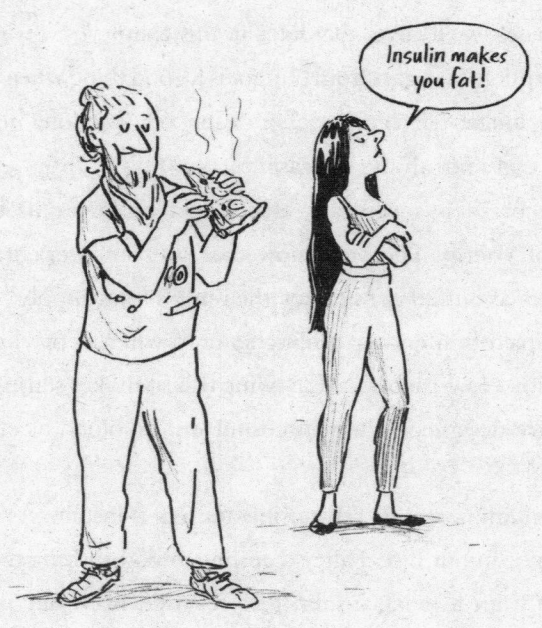

using the word 'insulin' with a dirty look on their face like they just smelt something foul. Insulin is not a dirty word! The fact it helps our body store fat is not something to be afraid of.

Does any of that help to explain just how important and normal the stimulation and production of insulin is? Less scary yet? It's almost as if we evolved with the consumption of carbohydrates in mind . . .

That might have felt like more science than you would have chosen to read, but it will help cut through the nutribollocks – I promise.

Ready to address some nonsense?

'CARBOHYDRATES AREN'T ESSENTIAL'

When used as an excuse to demonise carbs, this statement is just stupid. The official term for an 'essential nutrient' is one that has to be eaten because the body can't make it on its own. Both protein and fat provide nutrients that meet that criteria, but carbohydrates don't, as glucose can be made from both protein and fat. As such, our bodies are technically able to survive without carbohydrates, but is that really what you're aiming for? Do you want to go through life just surviving? Doing the bare minimum to function? This is an incredibly reductionist approach; food is far more than just fuel.

Picture the food that makes you feel most at home. Maybe it's the meal your parents used to make on a weekend, or the one that you and your partner make together. Try picturing your favourite meal as a child. You don't remember the breakdown of carbs, fats and protein because they aren't important.

If you want to only eat what is 'essential' for your body to function, you might as well only drink meal-replacement shakes. That was sarcasm by the way; please don't do that. It would be a miserable existence.

If you don't enjoy eating carbs and you honestly and truly feel better without including them in your diet, that's fine. I'm not here to make rules around food in either direction. If, however, you've been convinced you shouldn't eat carbs because they 'aren't essential', please know that this is complete nonsense.

'CARBS MAKE YOU FAT'

No, they don't.

In order to address this, we need to talk about something known as the carbohydrate-insulin model of ob*sity, something first suggested in 2006[76] by Dr Robert Lustig, an American doctor who has since published several anti-sugar books. He claims that because insulin stimulates fat storage and reduces fat metabolism, carbohydrates are the biggest reason why people gain weight and therefore we shouldn't be eating them.

It seems potentially logical at first glance, especially as the claims around insulin sound like good science, but you'll be glad to hear it starts to fall apart when you do a little digging.

One of the best ways this has been tested is in weight-loss studies where one group is given a low-carb diet and the other a low-fat one. This is important as dietary fat doesn't stimulate insulin release, but protein does, so the best way to isolate the effect of insulin is by keeping protein and calories equal between groups. For the carbohydrate-insulin model to be correct, the low-carb diet should result in more fat loss than the low-fat one. Not to give the game away right at the beginning, but the problem is that it doesn't.

A systematic review and meta-analysis (remember to use the cheat sheet for these terms on pages 11 and 12 if you need to) in 2017 looked at 32 studies comparing weight loss between low-carb and low-fat diets[77]. The low-carb diet didn't show *any* meaningful benefit in body fat loss or daily energy expenditure.

One incredibly well-controlled metabolic ward study even found that those on the low-fat diet lost slightly *more* weight, despite having higher insulin levels[78].

The presence of insulin doesn't override the fact that we only store extra energy as fat if we *have* extra energy. We wouldn't function very well otherwise! If the carbohydrate-insulin model was true it would also mean that carbohydrates should lead to more weight gain than any other macronutrient. Fortunately, we can test that quite easily. There aren't actually that many studies on this topic (overfeeding studies tend to be done less frequently than restriction studies), but three relevant ones exist[79–81]. As expected, *none* of them found that overfeeding with carbohydrates led to more body fat gain than overfeeding with dietary fat.

As the well-respected researcher Stephan Guyenet PhD succinctly puts it, 'Clearly, an excess calorie of fat gets into fat tissue as effectively as an excess calorie of carbohydrate, regardless of their effects on insulin.'[82]

What about countries that eat lots of carbs?

If carbs truly are the culprit for weight gain then countries eating the most should have a higher average body weight. Sounds logical?

Let's take a look at Japan. They have one of the highest consumptions of carbs of all the OECD countries (Organisation for Economic Co-operation and Development). White rice is a staple at pretty much every meal (including breakfast), yet despite this they still have the lowest ob*sity rate[83]. The official Japanese Food Guide Spinning Top recommends five to six vegetable dishes and five to seven grain dishes per day[84], something that would *horrify* the low-carb evangelists.

What about in the US? Between 1999 and 2016 the overall carbohydrate intake fell from 52.5 per cent to 50.5 per cent, with the intake from added sugar decreasing from 16.4 per cent to 14.4 per cent. Intake of whole grains actually increased, but not enough to stop the decrease in overall carbs[85]. Despite all this reduction in insulin stimulation, average body size has been continuing to increase[86].

Now, obviously, analysing increases in body size is far more complex than simply looking at carbohydrate intake. I'm not negating that. However, it makes it even harder to blame carbs and insulin when we're faced with the reality that declining carbohydrate intake is corresponding globally with increases in body fat. Sounds like it was never the carbohydrates after all!

It's not just little old me that's saying this either by the way. In 2015 the Department of Health and the Food Standards Agency in the UK commissioned the Scientific Advisory Committee on Nutrition to examine the latest evidence on the links between consumption of carbohydrates and a range of health outcomes[87]. They concluded that higher-carbohydrate diets not only had no effect on overall body weight, but also had no effect on total fat mass or waist-to-hip ratio.

Why might low-carb diets seem better?

Lots of people believe, from personal experience, that a low-carb diet must be the best due to the initial weight loss seeming more pronounced. This is due to the body first using up its stores of glycogen in order to maintain blood glucose levels, seeing as there aren't enough carbs being eaten to maintain it the normal way. Glycogen is stored as a hydrated form, with three to four parts water, so when converted back into glucose this water is lost. The initial big drop on the scales with a low-carb diet is simply a loss of water weight[88].

When challenged properly on the fact that carbs don't make you fat, many will change tack and claim that they never actually meant *all* carbs, only the refined ones. You may have been reading along and wondering if there's a distinction between certain car-bohydrates when it comes to weight gain. It's a fair question, so let's have a specific look at sugar, shall we?

'SUGAR MAKES YOU FAT'

As this is such a pervasive sentiment, one that is almost impossible to escape from if you spend any time online, we should probably go through it in a little more detail.

Sugar isn't unique when it comes to energy balance either. If you increase the amount of sugar in your diet while keeping overall calories the same, predictably, weight doesn't change. A systematic review and meta-analysis[89] looked at 12 different stud-ies that all swapped dietary sugars for either fat or protein and found *no* difference in weight. Having said that, the same review looked at ten different studies that *didn't* control for calories and found that a higher sugar intake correlated with an overall greater consumption of food and weight gain.

So, why is that? There are three simple reasons why increasing sugar intake might lead to people eating more overall:

1. Sugar is highly palatable (makes food taste great).
2. Sugar is calorie-dense.
3. Sugar isn't particularly filling.

Add these together and you can see why a diet high in sugar might lead to overeating. We can acknowledge this without choosing to demonise sugar by saying that any amount of sugar 'causes people to get fat'.

Sugar and processed food

One of the biggest sources of added sugar intake is often the consumption of processed food. Let's look at a recent trial[90] that compared people's eating habits between an ultra-processed and an unprocessed diet. Ultra-processed in this context is defined as being made 'mostly of cheap . . . sources of dietary energy and nutrients plus additives, using a series of processes' and high in 'fat, refined starches, free sugars' and are 'poor sources of protein'[91]. This included things like fried chicken nuggets, pre-made sandwiches, sausages, crisps and packet ravioli. Those taking part were allowed to eat as much or as little as they wanted until they were full. Those given the ultra-processed diet ended up consuming roughly an extra 500kcal a day over the two weeks and gained weight compared to those given the unprocessed one. The study matched the two diets for both sugar and macronutrients, indicating that it was the processed nature *itself* responsible for the overconsumption rather than any specific nutritional difference.

We know that ultra-processed diets can lead to people eating more and we know that high amounts of sugars are present in ultra-processed foods. As mentioned above though, so are high amounts of fat and lower amounts of protein[92]. Fat has actually been shown to be the main common denominator (not refined carbs) when it comes to hyper-palatable foods[93], so maybe fat is actually the culprit leading to overconsumption here . . . or maybe weight gain is too complex to be trying to put the blame on one macronutrient.

Protein has been shown to be the most satiating macronutrient[94] (the feeling of fullness), so maybe the lack of protein associated with a diet high in refined carbs leads to overconsumption as a result of less satiety . . . *or maybe weight gain is too complex to be trying to put the blame on one macronutrient.*

Are you sensing a theme?

Before we move on it's really important to note that demonising ultra-processed food isn't the answer here either; many rely on it to feed themselves and their families. Being able to cook fresh food from scratch is a massive socio-economic privilege that not everyone has access to (see page 36).

Let's look at sugary drinks

What about drinking sugar rather than eating it? Researchers argue about this quite a lot, partly due to the fact that the vast majority of research specifically looking at sugary drinks and weight gain hasn't actually been done very well[95]. The couple of research papers that *are* of good quality give completely different conclusions; one states that there would be no effect of reducing the intake of sugary drinks on body weight[96] and the other is confident that they promote weight gain[97] .

Other research has shown that, in general, drinks aren't as filling as food[98,99] especially those without any protein or fat[100]. Studies comparing drinking water and sugary drinks during meals showed that both groups of participants still ate exactly the same amount[101], indicating that the consumption of sugar-sweetened beverages may result in extra energy on top of a regular diet.

Would I use the phrase 'sugar-sweetened drinks make you fat'? No, because there are a multitude of other socio-economic factors associated with their consumption that play a factor. Weight gain is complex (see pages 51–52). Would I, as a doctor, advise against their overconsumption? Yes, but that's mainly due to the non-weight related health impact of added sugars in the diet, from a potential increase in heart disease[102] to your likelihood of a mounting dental bill.

Good news! We are actually eating less sugar

How many of you have been told that our sugar intake is rising and it's therefore no surprise that we're gaining weight? This final argument is just categorically untrue, no matter how you look at it.

The UK government has been collecting household food and

drink data since 1974 – let me give you an overview. Our intake of sugars, jams, biscuits, cakes and pastries has fallen, leading to an overall reduction in total sugar intake by around 17.5 per cent in the last 20 years[103–105]. That data doesn't fit the wellness narrative though does it? Although we're still eating too much, sugar intake has been falling ever since the 70s and doesn't correlate at all with body weight at a population level, yet you'd never know it from the overwhelming rhetoric that implies otherwise.

While sugar *is* energy-dense and certainly able to add to overall energy intake, the evidence doesn't support the notion that it's causative of weight gain. Those who adamantly insist that it does almost always have a low-carb diet book to sell you.

'DIABETICS SHOULDN'T EAT CARBS'

If you're someone living with diabetes you may be surprised to hear me say this, but you don't *have* to cut out carbs unless you specifically want to. No one should ever be automatically prescribed a certain way of eating unless they are allergic to something. You have a relationship with food. Food is more than just fuel; it's culture, memories, celebration, emotion . . . and choice.

Diabetes is a group of metabolic disorders characterised by high blood glucose levels. Type 1 is when the pancreas doesn't produce enough insulin and type 2 usually starts with the body becoming resistant to it.

Without any insulin (type 1), blood glucose levels skyrocket as they can't be moved into the cells. This results in a triad of uncontrollable hunger, excessive thirst and increased volume of urination, and if left untreated can progress to what's known as diabetic ketoacidosis (DKA). With the body grasping to find energy to use, there is an uncontrolled release of something called ketones as the body breaks down fat cells instead. These ketones actually make the blood more acidic and without medical intervention it ends up being fatal. We'll touch on this stuff again later in Chapter 6 when talking about the ketogenic diet.

On the other hand, insulin resistance (type 2) means that the body is less responsive to it, resulting in the blood glucose levels sitting chronically higher than they should be. If left unmanaged this can lead to complications such as high blood pressure, worsening vision, nerve damage to the feet and skin infections.

For someone *without* diabetes, no matter what's eaten or how inactive they are, blood glucose levels almost *always* stay within a normal range. With this no longer being the case for someone living with diabetes it can be really beneficial to find a way of life that improves the outcome of having a chronic disease. Food can play a part in that.

Seeing as carbohydrates have the biggest impact on blood glucose levels compared to other macronutrients, people with diabetes who cut them completely from their diet will often find they have better blood glucose control. This can lead to stories being shared and others being told to do the same, but every choice in life has to be weighed up with a knowledge of risk.

Removing *all* carbohydrates brings with it the added complication of an incredibly restrictive diet negatively impacting your relationship with food. This can be in the form of added stress around food shopping, thinking of carbs as 'bad' or the lack of flexibility when out and about. All of these can have much more impact than you'd expect.

Lack of carbs often leads to a loss of beneficial nutrients such as fibre and can also lower energy levels, making it harder for people to exercise, both of which would normally have the potential to *improve* insulin resistance in the context of type 2 diabetes. The final issue that often gets swept under the rug is the risk for those restricting carbohydrates to experience harmful increases in cholesterol levels[106]. We'll talk about that in the next chapter.

I still remember an incident as a newly qualified doctor dealing with an unconscious, barely breathing patient with type 1 diabetes. She'd been brought into A&E with incredibly low blood glucose levels after accidentally giving herself too much insulin. Fifteen minutes later, after administering glucose into one of her veins, she was sitting up, smiling and eating a biscuit. Sugar can be life-saving for those with diabetes and demonising carbohydrates doesn't help matters at all.

So, if you don't have to remove carbohydrates *completely*, is there any benefit to *reducing* them? For many with diabetes, a lower-carb diet can definitely help with the management of blood glucose. It would be disingenuous for me to pretend otherwise. The important thing to note here is that there are ways to do that without going to an extreme and demonising them unnecessarily. If you're living with diabetes you can respect the impact that carbohydrates have while still including them in your diet. For example, choosing wholegrain, complex carbohydrates that have less of an impact on blood glucose is a good start.

Now, if you are reading this and living with diabetes, it's not my job to give you individual dietary advice in this book – that wouldn't be sensible. There are however some general things that are advised by both the NHS and many different diabetic organisations that I'll include below:

- consume carbohydrates as part of a balanced meal with sources of both protein and fat
- choose wholegrain sources when available
- increase your vegetable intake
- increase sources of fibre
- increase your protein intake
- try to minimise refined carbohydrates and simple sugars that have the potential to impact your blood glucose levels to a greater extent

These are suggestions not rules; this advice is not based around restriction but *inclusion*. As always with the management of a chronic condition, make sure that you speak to your doctor and the people involved in your healthcare.

'SUGAR CAUSES TYPE 2 DIABETES'

No it doesn't. There are many complex genetic and environmental factors that can increase the risk of type 2 diabetes, but sugar is not a cause.

It's not uncommon to assume that because type 2 diabetes is

characterised by having high blood sugar, consuming sugar must be the culprit. These two are not the same and by the end of this chapter you should have a better understanding why.

Many people lump type 1 and type 2 together as just 'diabetes' when they really shouldn't. In type 1 diabetes, the beta cells of the pancreas that produce insulin are destroyed by a person's own immune system – this is usually a result of a genetic predisposition with an environmental trigger such as a viral infection. This results in little to no insulin production. What you eat has absolutely nothing to do with it.

Type 2 diabetes usually starts with the cells of the body becoming less responsive to insulin (insulin resistance). At the same time there is a progressive loss of pancreatic beta cell function, which can eventually lead to a loss of insulin production. There are many different things that can increase the risk of insulin resistance and hence developing type 2 diabetes, including:

- distribution of body fat
- genetics/family history of diabetes
- ethnicity
- being of older age
- low levels of physical activity
- low dietary fibre intake
- PCOS (polycystic ovary syndrome)
- high blood pressure
- chronic stress
- sleep deprivation

This isn't an exhaustive list. Type 2 diabetes is incredibly multifactorial, combining genetic, environmental and lifestyle factors. Out of the gate it's clear to see that it would be incorrect to blame its development on any single factor like sugar.

A discussion about body fat

I'd like to talk briefly about the link between body fat and type 2 diabetes, as this is something that not only members of the public, but qualified doctors, tend to misrepresent. Increased body fat has the potential to lead to insulin resistance, but it's very dependent on *where* that fat is on the body. As mentioned earlier (see page 48), fat can be thought of as an endocrine organ due to its ability to produce numerous different things such as hormones and growth factors. Its function and activity change depending on its location within the body and as such, distribution of body fat can have a big impact on the risk of developing type 2 diabetes.

The best evidence we have is that increased visceral fat (around the organs) has the biggest harmful impact on insulin resistance[21], with subcutaneous fat (under the skin) around the abdomen coming in second. Subcutaneous fat in other locations, such as the hips and thighs, may even actually be protective[22]. One of the reasons why ethnicity can have an impact on type 2 diabetes risk is due to these differences in fat distribution[107].

Not only do our genetics play a major role in where we store fat but there are also many lifestyle factors that can contribute. Lack of exercise, poor sleep quality, lack of dietary fibre and chronic stress are all positively associated with fat being stored viscerally.

Increasing overall body weight *can* correlate with visceral fat, but it's not a good measure. As we already covered (see page 48), almost a third of people with a 'normal' weight are actually metabolically unhealthy and at increased risk for developing type 2 diabetes[18].

It's far too common to hear people stigmatise others for their weight under the guise of, 'I'm just concerned about your health . . . what about your risk of diabetes?' This concern trolling has become the go-to justification for weight stigma, as it's thought of as something that can't be argued against. It's inaccurate and should be challenged.

I haven't forgotten this section is meant to be about sugar, but it would have felt lacking had I not talked about the elephant in the room first. Let's now move on to the sweet stuff.

Surely sugar makes diabetes worse though?

It makes me sad when I hear people say they can't eat an item of food because they 'don't want to get diabetes' . . . it's always something stereotypical like a doughnut or sweets that are known to contain a fair amount of sugar. Regrettably, I used to think along the same lines as well. I'm not sure if that was my medical school's fault or some other reason, but I'm inclined to believe it's the former as I've found myself correcting colleagues on the issue as well.

The main argument, often used by self-identified 'low-carb' doctors, is that stimulating too much insulin with food leads to our cells becoming resistant to it. You might be surprised to hear this, but there is actually no evidence at all for this being true. *None*. The release of insulin as a response to eating food, including sugar, is normal and won't lead to insulin resistance. High-carbohydrate diets are actually associated with *improved* insulin sensitivity in normal individuals[108]!

Another argument is that it's actually a certain *type* of sugar, specifically fructose, that causes type 2 diabetes by leading to an increase in visceral fat. This is the type of sugar found in fruit and high-fructose corn syrup, the latter being most commonly used in the US in sugar-sweetened drinks and processed food. The evidence for this claim isn't as good as they'd like you to believe it is, with most of the studies having been performed in rodents (remember, you are not a mouse).

The studies with fructose that exist in humans are all in the context of excess energy intake[109]. Excess energy *can* be stored as visceral fat, but this would be the case no matter what food was being looked at[110]. This isn't unique to fructose and certainly isn't proof that it causes type 2 diabetes.

At the end of all that, is there enough evidence to be able to state that sugar causes type 2 diabetes? No. Which is the reason why you won't find any respected organisation or government saying that it does . . . only those who want to demonise sugar intake.

'SUGAR IS AS ADDICTIVE AS COCAINE'

Another absurd claim thrown around in order to convince people to avoid sugar is that it's addictive . . . like 'hard drugs' addictive. The first time this idea became mainstream (that I'm aware of) was in 2014's terrible nutrition movie *Fed Up* (movie is a much more accurate word than documentary here). About thirty seconds into the trailer[111] an image plays on the screen showing two near-identical functional MRI brain scans side-by-side with the labels 'SUGAR' and 'COCAINE' underneath them. Dr Robert Lustig, known for proposing the carbohydrate–insulin model and writing multiple books demonising 'toxic' sugar, then narrates: 'your brain lights up with sugar just like it does with cocaine or heroin; you're going to become an addict!' Oddly enough he seems to forget to mention that playing with puppies also lights up the same areas of the brain . . . but I guess that would only have been relevant if he was selling books arguing against pet ownership.

In 2017 the addiction idea got more airtime after a research review by James DiNicolantonio was published in the *British Journal of Sports Medicine*[112]. In it he claims that sugar addiction is not only real, but should be classified as a disease. Let's address why this is misguided.

One of the claims in the review is that animal behavioural studies show that sugar is an addictive substance. Sounds damning. Now, under certain conditions, it is true that rats can be made to develop addiction-like behaviours with respect to sugar[113]. Let's look at what those conditions actually were. First, only rats that show a preference for sugar are used[114], as not all of them do. Second, a feeding schedule is used that deliberately deprives the rodents of food for prolonged periods of time (in some instances for 16 hours[115]). This way, when they are finally allowed to eat, the rodents are more likely to exhibit addiction-like behaviours, such as bingeing and reported withdrawal anxiety. I'm pretty sure we'd all act the same way if we were starved against our will without knowing why it was happening.

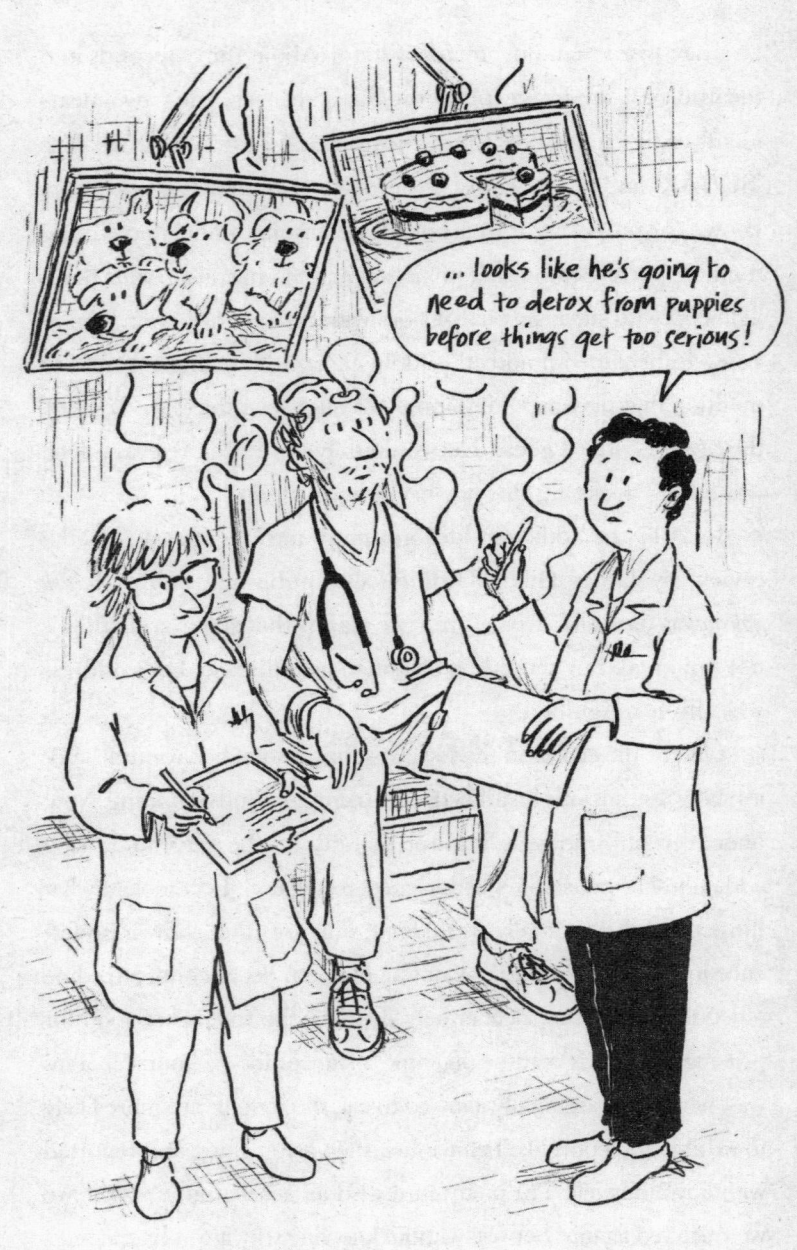

It's important to note that none of these behaviours in rats have ever been shown to occur without these restriction periods[114], indicating that the restriction is the problem, not the sugar. This is also backed up by research that shows fasting itself can increase the incidence of binge-eating and bulimic pathology[116] in humans. True addiction has both psychological and physical components; rats are not a perfect model for humans on either of these factors.

Sweet foods are often preferred by those with binge-eating disorders[117], something DiNicolantonio also uses as an argument for sugar being addictive. Sugar is ubiquitously demonised by diet culture, giving it extra psychological weight when it comes to a binge episode. I'd argue that it's not the supposed addictive quality of sugar that's the issue, but the years of restricting it out of fear of weight gain. It always greatly concerns me when those who have written diet books show themselves to have very little insight into the complexities of eating disorders.

The last point made by the review is the same as the propaganda film I mentioned at the beginning: both sugar and cocaine interact with the same reward system in the brain. The big problem with using this to argue for sugar being addictive is that many things interact with this same reward system (such as puppies and hugs) but only drugs of abuse have the potential to hijack them. Sugar does not. Sugar not only has *no ability* to elicit physical withdrawal symptoms, but the psychological symptoms pale in comparison as well. Habit-forming is *not* the same as addiction and sugar simply doesn't fit the criteria for things like dependency or withdrawal.

Thomas Sanders, an emeritus professor of nutrition and dietetics at King's College London, summed it up perfectly: '[it's] *absurd* to suggest that sugar is addictive like hard drugs'[118].

'ARTIFICIAL SWEETENERS ARE HARMFUL'

It's really common to be afraid of something that's been labelled 'artificial', seeing as we tend to fear what we don't understand.

Artificial sweeteners are substances that taste sweet (shocker, I know) but provide little to no energy or nutrition. Like everything added to food, they have been subject to rigorous testing in order to work out whether they are safe for human consumption. The good news is that they most certainly are.

To give you context as to just how safe artificial sweeteners are, let's have a look at how many cans of Diet Coke you would have to drink before the aspartame (one of the main commercial sweeteners) in them becomes a problem. The rough estimate is about *1,900 cans* in a day.

The food standards agencies responsible for how much of a particular food additive can be used at one time are incredibly cautious. So much so that they've set the recommended daily intake at less than 100 times the toxic dose, meaning that the amount you end up actually consuming is minuscule. Artificial sweeteners are the most widely researched food additives we have and are *incredibly* safe[119].

Let's rapid-fire through some of the other claims about why artificial sweeteners are a problem:

- 'Artificial sweeteners damage your gut microbiome.'
  The majority of evidence for this is, once again, in
  rodents. There are a few studies in humans suggesting
  that they might be able to change the bacterial
  makeup of the gut, but how long it lasts for and
  whether that's actually damage or not is difficult to
  tell[120]. Overconsumption of some specific sweeteners
  can lead to flatulence and loose stools so there may be
  a smidge of truth to it.

- 'Artificial sweeteners cause type 2 diabetes.' Studies
  in rodents suggested that they might increase insulin
  resistance by interfering with the gut microbiome;
  however human studies haven't shown this to be
  the case[121]. Remember, you are not a mouse. The
  argument is often that sweeteners trigger insulin release
  due to the brain recognising the sweet taste. However,
  studies are very inconsistent with this and overall fail to
  show any effect on blood glucose levels[122].

- 'Aspartame causes headaches.' You might find this
  surprising, but this one hasn't been shown to be true
  either. Research conducted decades ago on people
  who reported getting headaches after consuming
  aspartame found that they were actually more likely to
  experience symptoms after being given a placebo[123].

- 'Artificial sweeteners cause cancer.' My friend recently
  reminded me that I used to believe this one as a
  teenager myself, but the good news is that it's not true
  at all. We'll talk about this later on (see page 218).

It's far too easy to find news articles reporting that artificial sweeteners are safe to consume because some recent study has shown that they don't cause weight gain. I know I'm repeating myself, but remember, weight and health are not the same thing. The fact that artificial sweeteners aren't a risk to your health has absolutely nothing to do with the number on the scales.

Make carbs great again

We need to stop letting wellness get away with demonising carbs. It damages people's relationship with food and fuels our phobia of weight gain.

I know that for some of you this chapter will have been particularly difficult. When it comes to that list of foods that we've decided are 'bad' and must be avoided, carbohydrates tend to feature right at the beginning. The fear of carbs can become so overwhelming that it controls every choice we make around food; it was this fear that fuelled my most disordered eating habits not that long ago. Eating is meant to be an enjoyable experience, one with pleasure, satisfaction and comfort. Carbohydrates should play a role in that.

If the above resonates, please take this as permission to let yourself eat carbs again. They are wonderful. Pop the kettle on and make yourself a cup of tea, grab a couple of chocolate biscuits and let's talk about the myths around dietary fat.

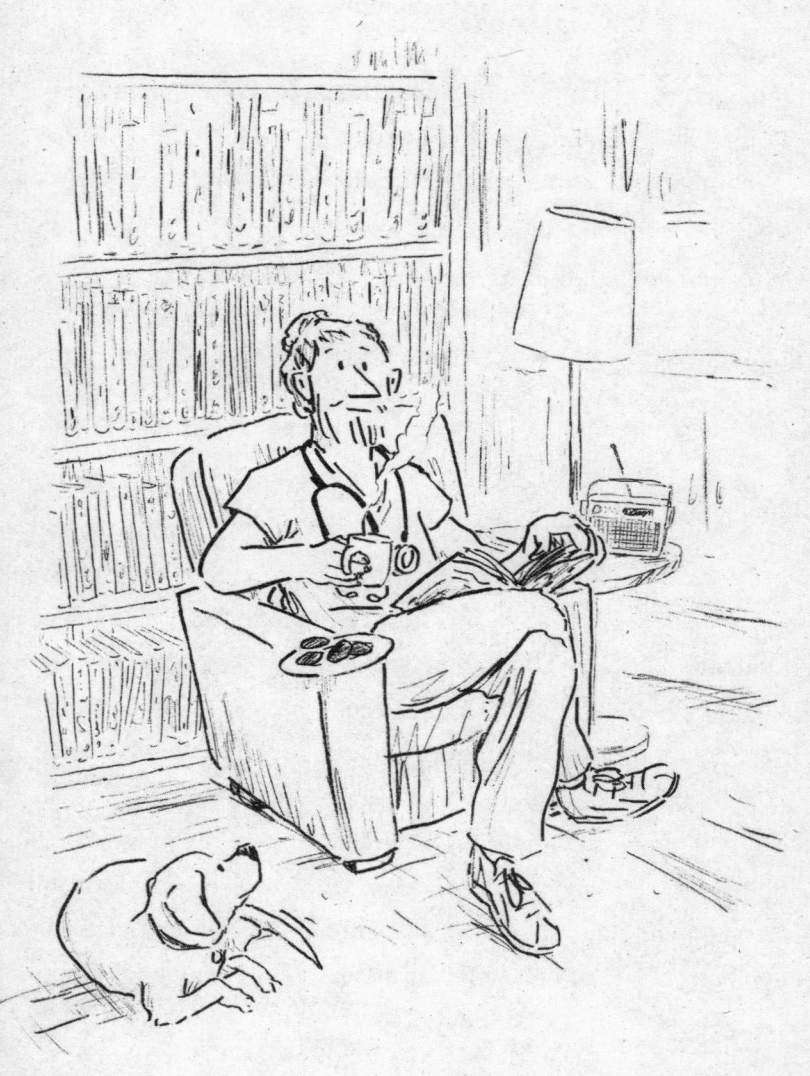

5.

IS EATING FAT BAD FOR YOU?

The misinformation around different types of dietary fat is one of the things that gets nutritional scientists the *most* riled up, as it tends to originate from doctors and scientists who should really know better. When you read headlines in the paper such as, 'Eating saturated fat is good for you: Doctors change their minds after 40 years,' please know that this simply isn't true. The last sentence should actually read '. . . a few rogue, low-carb, saturated fat-denialist doctors change their mind in order to sell books.'

In this chapter we'll look at a range of things, from the nonsense surrounding saturated fat to the confusion around cholesterol and eggs, and this new obsession with demonising vegetable oils. Before all that though, let's start with why fat is so important in our diet to begin with.

Why we need to eat fat

Just like we talked about with carbohydrates, fat in our diet is really important. It helps us absorb micronutrients such as fat-soluble vitamins (A, D, E and K) and is used by our body for a whole host of different functions, from forming parts of our cells to making hormones. Fat can also be used for energy; the extent to which this occurs depends on the type of cell it's being used by.

On top of all that, fat is what makes food taste amazing. Toast? Boring. Toast with butter? Now you're talking! We have to talk about the nutrients in food a fair bit in this book in order to address the slew of nutribollocks, but don't forget that food is so much more than just nutrients.

The science of fat and heart health

The fat we eat gets broken down by our gut into smaller compounds called triglycerides. These are then classified as either saturated or unsaturated, with food containing different ratios of each. You will have almost certainly heard of cholesterol; we get some from our food but the majority is made by our liver. We will talk more about that in a bit.

A good way of distinguishing if the fat in food is mainly saturated or unsaturated is whether the fat is solid at room temperature. Butter and coconut oil? Solid and mostly saturated fat. Olive oil? Liquid and mostly unsaturated. There are exceptions to this rule but overall, it's a pretty good one.

After the dietary fat is absorbed in the gut it's transported by the blood around the body to where it is then either used or stored. Seeing as fat and water don't mix particularly well, neither triglycerides nor cholesterol are able to float along in the blood by themselves, so in order to be transported they are packaged up into what are called lipoproteins. There are four main types to be aware of:

- Chylomicrons – these transport triglycerides around the body from the intestine after a meal.
- Very low-density lipoproteins (VLDL) – these transport triglycerides made by the liver.
- Low-density lipoproteins (LDL) – these carry cholesterol away from the liver to parts of the body where it is needed.
- High-density lipoproteins (HDL) – these carry cholesterol back to the liver for recycling and/or disposal.

Researchers first noticed that there seemed to be an association between high total cholesterol levels in the blood and cardiovascular disease back in the 1930s[124]. When cholesterol is high it can be deposited on the walls of our arteries and form what is known as atherosclerotic plaque. As it progresses, and the artery gets narrower, this plaque can get in the way of the flow of blood and lead to a heart attack or stroke, depending on which vessels are the problem. As the years went by it was shown that having high LDL and low HDL was the worst combination for cardiovascular risk[125,126], seeing as LDL carried cholesterol to where it had potential to get stuck and HDL took it back to the liver.

Let's talk about LDL first as it gets mentioned a lot in this discussion. We know that reducing LDL levels is the most reliable way of improving cardiovascular risk[127]. Statins, the most common type of medication that we use to reduce LDL when it's high, can have brilliant results in terms of reducing someone's risk of heart attacks and strokes[128].

It was also thought that by actively increasing HDL we could also reduce risk, but medication designed to do just that unfortunately hasn't shown any benefit[129]. Having a low HDL is still considered to be a bad thing when assessing risk[130,131], but increasing it can't undo the negative effect of a high LDL, so we focus on reducing the latter. Be aware that those who spread misinformation when it comes to diet and cardiovascular risk often use this complexity to cause confusion and sow seeds of doubt.

So, if reducing LDL is the goal, which it is, what do we know when it comes to our diet that can help us do that?

- ***Avoid trans fats[132]***

  These are formed when vegetable oils are partially hydrogenated for use in margarine and other processed food. The good news is that since we found out their consumption increased LDL, changing regulations have reduced them considerably from the food supply in Western Europe; it's actually quite hard to find any spreads in the supermarket with them anymore. Several countries across the world (including the US) have even banned industrially produced trans fats from the food supply altogether.

- ***Reduce your saturated fat intake[133]***

  Research has not only shown us that a high saturated fat intake increases LDL[67], but also that reducing consumption has the ability to lower both LDL and our cardiovascular risk[134]. The UK guidelines recommend sticking to less than 30g a day for men or 20g a day for women[135]. Note: the saturated fat from most dairy is an exception to this rule. Milk, cream, cheese and yoghurt don't cause LDL to increase[136], but saturated fat from butter does. I'll explain why later on in this chapter.

- ***Increase your dietary fibre[137]***

   Increasing fibre in the diet has been shown to reduce levels of LDL and with it cardiovascular disease risk[138]. The guidance for adults is to get at *least* 30g a day[87].

There are also non-diet lifestyle factors that can reduce LDL, such as exercise, stopping smoking and reducing alcohol intake. It's important to reiterate that although food and lifestyle can have an impact on cardiovascular risk by altering your cholesterol profile, they have their limitations. If your levels are high enough that your doctor has prescribed you medication such as a statin, don't think you can automatically cheat the need for it by following the points above. It's both. Not either/or. Have I mentioned that food isn't medicine?

Enough build-up though . . . shall we look at some of the bad science that the saturated fat and cholesterol denialists use to spread their misinformation? Are you ready?

'SATURATED FAT DOESN'T INCREASE CARDIOVASCULAR RISK'

If I had to choose just one thing for you to be clear on by the end of this whole chapter it would be the following statement:

> 'A diet high in saturated fat is undeniably bad for your cardiovascular risk.'

When it comes to food and disease the link between saturated fat consumption and cardiovascular risk is one of the strongest we have. Now, that doesn't mean you need to be *afraid* of it. You just need to have respect for, and have an understanding of, the impact that it can have. The misinformation needs to be replaced with information.

A wide range of different studies over the last 70 years have categorically shown us that a high saturated fat intake increases LDL levels[67]. We also know, without a shadow of a doubt, that increasing LDL causes cardiovascular disease[139]. This is enough by itself, but to tie it all up with a neat little bow: it's been shown that by reducing saturated fat intake we can actually reduce the risk of cardiovascular events by up to 17 per cent[134]. Interestingly, it's not only the reduction of saturated fat that's beneficial but what we end up replacing it with; the most benefit coming from unsaturated fats such as those found in oily fish and olive oil[140].

With all of that being widely accepted throughout the scientific community, you may be wondering why people are creating misinformation around the topic. It's a good question and a very important one.

The majority of the saturated fat denialists promote a low-carb, high-fat diet in some way, shape or form. This isn't a coincidence; it's much easier to justify eating a diet that contains way more fat than usual if saturated fat doesn't matter. Now, it's definitely *possible* to eat a high-fat diet without automatically consuming lots of saturated fat, but with research showing that these diets consistently increase LDL[106] I'd argue that this isn't happening. With heart disease one of the leading causes of death globally[141], we need to stop promoting diets that contribute to it!

You won't be surprised to hear that most of these denialists sell their theories in the form of diet books . . . isn't it interesting how money always seems to encourage wilful ignorance? Take one of the most infamous denialists in the UK, Dr Aseem Malhotra. His book, *The Pioppi Diet*, claims to help you lose weight and reverse type 2 diabetes by cutting out all carbs and eating lots of fat, sold with the authority bias of him actually being a cardiologist. Let's take it apart.

Pioppi is a small Italian fishing village that is widely recognised as the home of the Mediterranean diet; a way of eating commonly regarded as the gold standard when it comes to health and life expectancy[142]. You'd think it would be pretty hard to screw up writing a diet book on it, yet it made the British Dietetic Association's annual list of celebrity diets to avoid back in 2018[143].

The traditional Mediterranean diet includes lots of fruits, vegetables, nuts, legumes, olive oil, bread, pasta, fish, yoghurt, cheese and some meat. In terms of macronutrients, it has a split of around 40 per cent fat, 20 per cent protein and 40 per cent carbohydrates . . . the latter of which *usually* makes it pretty hard to fit in with the low-carb narrative. Malhotra's solution? Just cherry-pick the parts that fit what he wants to say and pretend that the rest isn't there. The book claims to tell the secrets of the village of Pioppi, but you won't find any normal pizza or pasta, just low-carb recipes made from cauliflower. If you can find me a traditional Italian grandma who doesn't roll around in laughter at the thought of making pizza from cauliflower, I'll eat my hat. He also tells the readers to start each day with a tablespoon of coconut oil in their coffee. Since when was coconut an Italian staple?!

A year earlier Malhotra co-produced a 'documentary' on Pioppi with the same message, only that time he stirred butter into his coffee alongside the coconut oil. Up until now this was just a nonsense fad diet, but that one coffee recipe *alone* contains your recommended daily intake of saturated fat. Don't worry though; in order to try to argue the potential heart disease problem away he included a dangerously misleading chapter in his book entitled, 'Saturated fat does not clog the arteries'.

Although members of the public who buy into this rhetoric may not see an *immediate* detrimental health effect, the undeniable long-term cardiovascular risks aren't a joke. This isn't something to be playing a game of chicken with.

Finally, we have the issue that Malhotra and many of the other saturated fat denialists like to demonise statins (a drug used *very* successfully to lower cardiovascular disease risk). A surge in media coverage about the topic a few years back directly resulted in people who were on these drugs deciding, against medical advice,

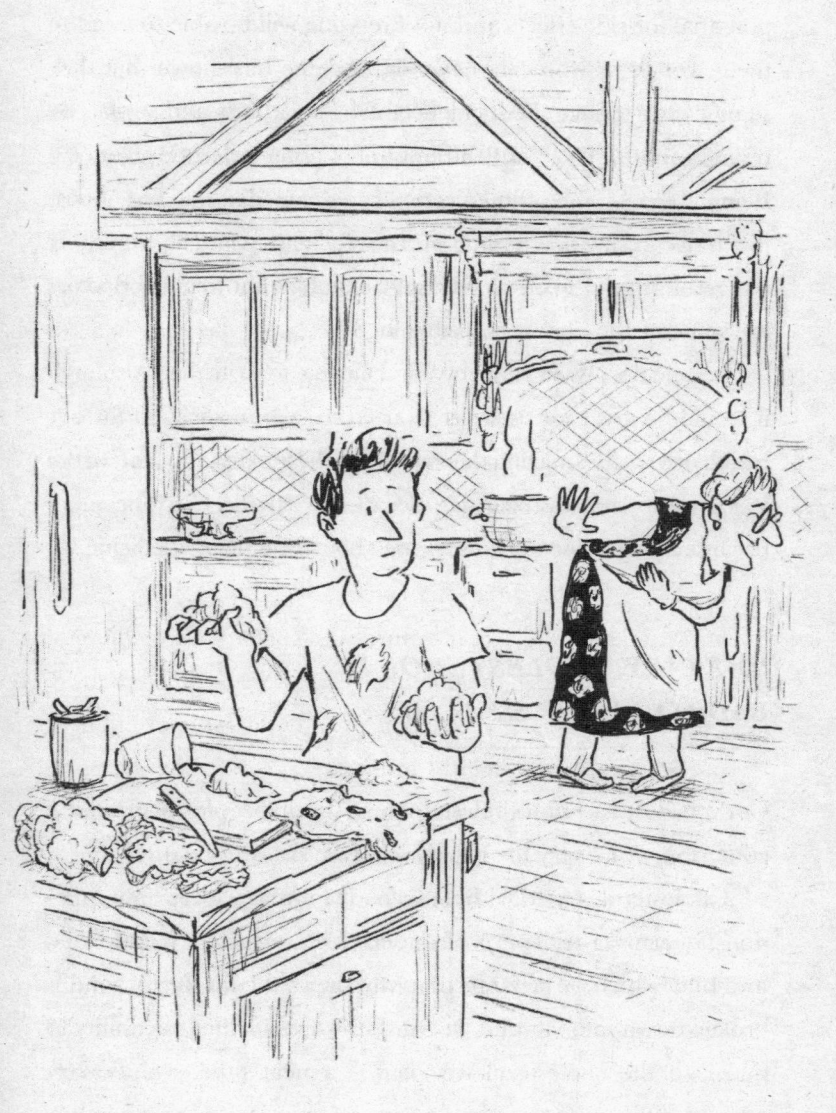

to stop taking them[144]. Like all medication, statins have the potential for side effects and not everyone will be able to tolerate them. For those who can, however, research has shown that they significantly reduce the incidence of heart attacks and strokes by reducing both LDL[128] and the amount of atherosclerotic plaque[145]. Being able to come off medication is a great thing . . . but choosing to stop taking it as a result of misinformation can be incredibly dangerous and it's completely unacceptable that medical doctors are some of the ones responsible for it.

. . . and no, I wasn't paid by 'Big Pharma' to write that. Although it would be great for us never to need to take medication for our health, it's pretty amazing that drugs like these exist for when we do. We need to stop disregarding decades of medical advancement because of some idealistic nonsense about food being medicine.

'DIETARY CHOLESTEROL IS BAD FOR YOUR HEALTH'

Conversations around cholesterol tend to trip people up and cause confusion, so let's try to simplify what we know to be true.

Cholesterol is used within our body for many important functions; it forms crucial parts of our cell membranes, gets converted into bile (which we need to properly digest the fat we eat) and is broken down into vitamin D. Our body actually has the ability to make all the cholesterol we need – a neat little evolutionary advantage from when animal products were less common in our diet. The majority of this production happens in the liver.

Ever since research started to show a relationship between overall cholesterol levels in the blood and heart disease risk, researchers have hypothesised that having too much cholesterol in the diet would mean higher levels of cholesterol in the blood[146]. It was a safe assumption to make at the time seeing as previous research had shown that feeding large amounts of cholesterol to animals led to atherosclerotic plaque formation.

However, we now know that this wasn't completely correct. First, a whole host of different factors affect how much dietary cholesterol is actually absorbed by our gut. Second, when the amount of cholesterol in our diet goes up it causes a reduction in how much our liver makes[147] and increases the amount produced as bile[148] (which ends up being excreted). In roughly two-thirds of the population these mechanisms are so good that dietary cholesterol has absolutely no impact on the amount of overall cholesterol in the blood[149].

The remaining third of the population don't compensate as well, leading to a very *slight* rise in overall cholesterol levels (both LDL and HDL). This sounds bad at first, but without going into too much complexity, this change has been shown *not* to have an effect on cardiovascular risk[150,151]. There may be a combined risk of very high dietary cholesterol on *top* of a diet high in saturated fat, but we know that the main driver of risk is the latter. The consumption of food high in cholesterol, such as eggs, has even been shown to be *beneficial* for heart health[152], suggesting that cholesterol by itself isn't worth worrying about.

Here's some added nuance. For the 0.5 per cent of the population who have the genetic condition called familial hyper-cholesterolaemia (where LDL levels are really high), the ability of

HDL to be protective is reduced[153], meaning that it may well be sensible to limit dietary cholesterol as a precaution. If this is you, discuss this with your doctor in person – a book should never count as personalised medical advice.

'DAIRY CAUSES INFLAMMATION'

Inflammation is often used as a buzzword. It's a good one too because it sounds scary – but what exactly does it mean?

When you have an injury or infection and a part of your body swells up and becomes hot, this is an example of inflammation playing an incredibly necessary and helpful part of our immune response. Like pretty much everything in our body, too much can be harmful and can play a role in conditions like rheumatoid arthritis and inflammatory bowel disease.

Do lifestyle factors like diet, exercise and sleep impact levels of inflammation? Sure, but that doesn't justify overly attributing blame to any individual element. When it comes to arguing that food causes or cures inflammation, the evidence is often very reductionist in nature. What I mean by that is instead of looking at food and eating patterns as a whole, people focus on specific nutrients in order to fit their argument. As we've been through already (see page 72), this is simply not how our diets work; we eat food, not nutrients.

It is often argued that dairy is 'pro-inflammatory' due to the saturated fat content, but there's more to it than first meets the eye. Although it's true that studies have shown saturated fat intake to be associated with low-grade inflammation[154], there is often no distinction drawn as to where that saturated fat comes from – a point that becomes very relevant when we're talking about dairy.

Dairy intake from milk, cream, cheese and yoghurt has *not* been shown to have a negative impact on cardiovascular risk and LDL[136] like other sources of saturated fat. They may even be beneficial[155]. The best theory as to why this is the case is that the combined effects of the structure of dairy nutrients prevent the saturated fat from being digested and absorbed properly by our gut.

Unfortunately, the churned nature of butter changes that nutrient structure, making it an exception to the dairy rule. The saturated fat in butter still has a negative effect on LDL, meaning that you should probably only be spreading it on your toast *or* stirring it into your coffee, not both. I'd recommend picking the toast.

Some of you might be asking why both the UK and US dietary guidelines still recommend consuming 'low-fat' dairy now that we've discovered the above. I would imagine there are a few factors at play here. First, the evidence is still relatively new in the grand scheme of things and it takes time for dietary guidelines to change . . . if it didn't, we'd be in a situation where changes would be made prematurely and subsequently reversed. This isn't great for public trust. Second, it's potentially difficult to communicate the differences between butter and other types of dairy at a population level without risking confusion. Third, our narrow-minded simplistic view of weight gain has led to public health advisors labelling full-fat dairy as a risk for making people fat, despite the fact that recent research shows the exact opposite to be true[156]. Frustratingly predictable, that last one.

Back to the original question of whether dairy causes

inflammation. A 2017 systematic review concluded that this is simply not true and as long as you don't have a milk allergy, dairy even appears to have a weak *anti*-inflammatory effect in the body[157]. The clinical significance of this stuff is highly debatable, meaning that dairy isn't going to be curing inflammatory conditions anytime soon, but you can rest assured that it most certainly isn't promoting it.

'EATING EGGS IS AS BAD AS SMOKING'

In 2017 a vegan propaganda movie called *What the Health* was released to the world. It contained a treasure trove of spurious

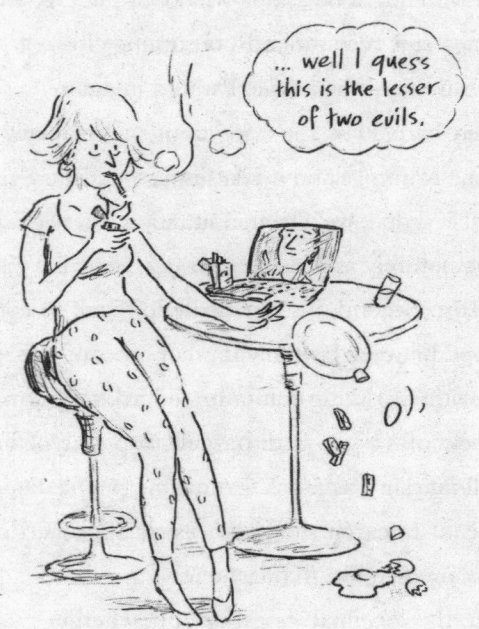

claims about nutrition, but one of the biggest was that eating one egg a day was as bad as smoking five cigarettes a day for life expectancy. Despite how ridiculous that sounds, it still gets quoted online to this day as a reason why we should all be avoiding eggs. The justification for this claim was a paper published in 2012 entitled, 'Egg yolk consumption and carotid plaque'[158]. Let's have a closer look at it.

The researchers looked at just over 1,200 patients attending hospital clinics for vascular disease prevention. They got them to fill out a questionnaire regarding their lifestyle (including how many egg yolks they consumed each week) and noted the size of the atherosclerotic plaque in one of the biggest arteries in the neck (the latter being a known predictor of cardiovascular disease risk). The conclusion they came to was that egg-yolk consumption increases carotid plaque size and therefore people at risk of cardiovascular disease should avoid eating egg yolks.

Now there's actually quite a few things wrong with that conclusion, but for the sake of time I'm just going to focus on the two biggest ones. I hope this will not only reassure you when it comes to egg consumption, but will also give you broader insight as to how data is sometimes manipulated in order to claim results that, when looked at properly, don't actually make much statistical sense.

To start with, we know that saturated fat intake has the biggest dietary impact on both cardiovascular risk and atherosclerotic plaque formation. This means that any research investigating diet and plaque size should include a measure of overall saturated fat intake . . . which this study conveniently chose not to. This makes it almost impossible to reach any sort of conclusions from the data.

The second problem with the study is the way they analysed the data. Instead of using how many egg yolks the patients consumed per week, they turned it into something that they called 'egg-yolk years'. They multiplied the egg yolks by how many years the patients had eaten eggs for. At first glance this approach seems okay, but let's test it. In a typical week I currently eat about five or six eggs. That number isn't always the same mind you; there are times in my life when I've not been eating them at all and other times when it's been an everyday breakfast item. With all of that variability, how would you accurately calculate my egg-yolk years? I have absolutely no idea what age I was when I first ate an egg, or how many eggs a week I would eat when I first left home and started buying food for myself. Trying to calculate the number of egg yolks someone has eaten over their lifetime just won't be accurate, and this inaccuracy is entirely unacceptable in a research context.

The researchers themselves would have known this, so the question remains: why did they choose to calculate it in this way? I believe the answer lies in the impact of age. Age is directly related to plaque size; the older we get, no matter how good our lifestyle is, plaque size and cardiovascular risk will increase. This means that, just like with saturated fat intake, the statistics have to account for age to make sure that it isn't causing the results.

Let me put it another way. If we asked the patients how many glasses of water they drank each day and multiplied this number by their age, we could get a value of 'water-glass years'. With age incorporated into the measure, we would then get results showing that drinking water increases cardiovascular risk, even though that's clearly ridiculous.

The researchers could have potentially fixed this problem by adjusting for age in the statistics, but they specifically argued that by using their measure of 'egg-yolk years' it meant that they couldn't. This is a) incredibly convenient, and b) not true at all. I would put good money on the fact that the only way they were able to find an association between eggs and plaque size was by doing it this way.

All this study actually showed was what we know already; as we age, atherosclerosis gets worse. The interpretation about egg-yolk consumption is complete nonsense.

Eggs are packed full of nutrients and can easily form part of a balanced diet. Studies have shown that because they only contain a small amount of saturated fat, even eating them over five times a week doesn't have a negative impact on cardiovascular risk[152,159]. As already discussed, we don't need to worry about their cholesterol content either. What's more, people who eat eggs are more likely to meet the recommendations for nutrients like choline, vitamin A and vitamin B12.

Just like the vast majority of the health documentary catalogue on Netflix, *What the Health* is a really terrible source of information when it comes to nutrition and diet. Best to avoid completely.

'VEGETABLE OIL IS TOXIC'

Vegetable oils (also known as seed oils) are obtained from the seed of a plant and mainly consist of unsaturated fat. The ones you'll have likely come across and might have in your kitchen are rapeseed (known as canola in the US), sunflower and sesame oil. Note: olives are technically a fruit (not a seed), so their oil doesn't fall into this category.

You will often find nonsense about these oils supposedly being 'toxic', or bad for you, coming from the saturated fat denialists. If they can convince you that vegetable oil causes heart disease, despite being very low in saturated fat, it makes it much easier to claim that saturated fat doesn't matter. It's in their best interest to spin this narrative as much as possible. However, because it's actually quite hard to argue that food high in mono- and polyunsaturated fat leads to heart disease, seeing as we have a plethora of evidence showing the exact opposite, they've had to be sneaky with their arguments.

The polyunsaturated fat in vegetable oil contains what are known as omega-3 and omega-6 fatty acids. Omega-3, also found in oily fish, has been linked to both brain health[160] and a potential reduction in heart disease risk[161,162]. It's hard to find anyone who argues against that. Rapeseed oil, in particular, is high in omega-3 and has a growing body of scientific evidence showing that it can reduce LDL and improve heart health[163]. It's not just olive oil that can be beneficial! Omega-6, on the other hand, despite also having been shown to decrease cardiovascular risk[164,165], has become the new scapegoat for apparently causing inflammation and disease.

The argument used against vegetable oils refers to the supposed inflammatory property of omega-6, with the claim being that the ratio of omega-6 to omega-3 is dangerously high in them. It's often accompanied by the spurious assumption that our ancestors didn't have chronic disease because they never used to eat as much omega-6 as we do. The more logical reason for that is because their life expectancy was too short for chronic disease to be a massive deal, but rational thinking isn't usually associated with denialism.

You'll be happy to hear that research has shown that this ratio of omega-6 to omega-3 means absolutely nothing when it comes to health[166]; vegetable oils can be great to include in your diet.

When you see someone take an incredibly complex phenomenon like chronic disease and attempt to reduce it down to just one nutrient, it's a good idea to question their reliability. One of the biggest proponents doing this is an American acupuncturist called Chris Kresser, who alongside being a saturated fat denialist and anti-vaxxer also sells books on how to follow the Paleo diet (a fad diet claiming to follow what our ancestors ate). Now without insinuating anything, I'm sure that fear-mongering omega-6 and blaming modern chronic disease on its consumption has absolutely no benefit to his book sales . . . none whatsoever. When you dig deeper into a lot of this kind of stuff you often find that those promoting the myths stand to gain the most from people believing them to be true.

It's not just Kresser with these views though. Google returns a whopping 8,440,000 results when you search 'omega 6 causes inflammation'. Should we be concerned even though the ratio mentioned earlier doesn't mean anything? The good news is that an inflammatory effect of omega-6 has never been shown in humans. In mice it has, but remember – you're not a mouse! Don't just take my word for it though; a systematic review[167] concluded that there is 'virtually no evidence . . . to show that addition of [omega-6] to the diet increases . . . inflammatory markers.'

For the nutrition geeks among you (who want to have even more ammo to argue against this stuff), the proposed mechanism by which omega-6 is meant to cause inflammation isn't valid either. The theory is that omega-6 is converted into a fatty acid called arachidonic acid, which in turn can be converted into molecules that promote inflammation . . . except the evidence shows that levels of arachidonic acid *don't* change after consuming omega-6[168]. Even if they did, arachidonic acid has also been shown to form *anti*-inflammatory molecules.

Finally, we also know that many foods high in omega-6 such as soy, nuts and seeds have all been shown to be good for our health. Be reassured – there's absolutely nothing inherently wrong with vegetable oil.

'COCONUT OIL IS A SUPERFOOD AND THE ONLY OIL YOU SHOULD USE'

Coconut oil has been endorsed by a multitude of wellness bloggers and celebrities. Whether it was as a result of Deliciously Ella using it in many of her recipes or The Body Coach Joe Wicks using it in his Instagram cooking videos, sales of coconut oil in the UK have risen from £1 million in 2014 to a whopping £26 million in 2018. After different medical associations started to express their concerns about people consuming so much, sales have started to fall, but the supposed health claims can still be found absolutely everywhere.

Coconut oil fits the wellness criteria to be labelled a 'superfood':

overly expensive, sounds natural, used by other cultures for decades before being 'discovered' by the West . . . Yet unlike goji berries, the Western use of coconut oil may actually be harming our health.

Coconut oil is 87 per cent saturated fat. As such, depending on how much you eat, its consumption has the potential to lead to a harmful increase in cholesterol levels. Proponents of its use will try to claim that it only leads to a rise in HDL cholesterol; however, a recent review of all the available research showed this simply not to be true. Coconut oil was shown to result in a substantial increase of LDL[169].

The thing is, this really shouldn't be that surprising. With two tablespoons of coconut oil containing 24g of saturated fat, it ends up being quite easy to go over the UK daily saturated fat guidelines of 20g for women and 30g for men.

Respect coconut oil and use it sparingly in dishes where it has the potential to impart flavour. Making it your main cooking oil is almost certainly a bad idea. Instead, use extra virgin olive oil seeing as that's been shown to actually *improve* heart health and, as such, is universally considered the healthiest source of fat[170] – back to that Mediterranean approach. Don't forget other ones like rapeseed as well; variety is always your friend!

'DIETARY GUIDELINES ON FAT ARE WRONG'

It's become common in recent years to blame government dietary guidelines for our rates of chronic disease and body size. The low-carb, high-fat advocates in particular claim that they demonise fat and encourage sugar consumption. Not only is it an incredibly lazy argument, but it's just simply nonsense.

In the US the first set of dietary 'goals' were published in 1977[171] and the following was recommended:

- increase your intake of fruit, vegetables and whole grains
- reduce overall fat consumption from 40 to 30 per cent of total energy intake
- reduce saturated fat intake to less than 10 per cent of total energy intake
- reduce sugar intake from 25 to 15 per cent of total energy intake
- reduce salt consumption to about 3g per day

Now, it's easy to nit-pick these guidelines, but let's be honest, increasing fruit, vegetables and whole grains while reducing saturated fat, sugar and salt isn't exactly controversial. The UK advice in 1983[172] was very similar but also included a specific instruction to increase total dietary fibre intake. What's impressive is that the vast majority of this advice still holds up today, with modern iterations of these guidelines really not having changed that much.

Frustratingly though, the overarching message of these guidelines back then was used to justify a craze for low-fat, with self-entitled weight-loss gurus playing a big role in encouraging the trend. By the end of the 1980s, fat-free egg white omelettes, low-fat yoghurts and boring iceberg lettuce salads (not to forget the low-fat dressing) were common in people's diets. We've come a long way since then, but we haven't left it behind completely yet.

The current culture of blaming nutritional guidelines for our health problems is not only incorrect but it detracts from the real issues. If everyone was able to follow the guidelines, we'd almost certainly see an improvement in overall health, but the majority of people who would most benefit aren't actually able to do so[173]. The guidelines don't matter when millions of people in the UK have limited access to affordable fresh fruit and vegetables and don't own a freezer. Food inequity has a bigger negative impact on our health than saturated fat or sugar intake ever could do.

Stop avoiding healthy fats

So, what's the take-home from this chapter when it comes to dietary fat? Let's put the low-fat craze of the late 20th century well and truly behind us and stop automatically buying the low-fat versions of things. Many of these tend to have high amounts of added sugar anyway. I'd much rather knowingly have my sugar in the form of cakes and other bakery goods than in a low-fat yoghurt!

Now, you do need to be sensible when it comes to your saturated fat intake, but don't let that mean you avoid the healthy* fats as well. We have evidence that suggests a reduced-fat diet is

---

* I usually don't like using the word 'healthy' when it comes to food as it can encourage the labelling of other foods as 'unhealthy' but I'm willing to make a slight exception if it reminds you about saturated fat. Just remember that no individual food is unhealthy in and of itself; quantity and context are everything!

worse than one including extra virgin olive oil when it comes to cardiovascular events like heart attacks and strokes[174], which sounds like a good reason not to avoid them to me!

Focus on getting more unsaturated fat into your diet from olive and rapeseed oil, nuts, seeds and sustainable fish . . . maybe even throw in some avocado toast? I know that a love of the latter has become a sarcastic joke as to why millennials don't have enough money to buy property, but we might as well embrace this particular stereotype!

6.

KETOGENIC DIETS AND INTERMITTENT FASTING

The low-carb Atkins diet boldly claimed to be the solution to weight loss and health in the 1960s. It wasn't. Now its inbred (should that be inbread? never mind . . .) cousin, the ketogenic diet, is implying that you just weren't restricting carbohydrates aggressively enough for it to work. It's always your fault, you see.

What does it mean to 'go keto'?

The ketogenic diet was originally developed by American doctor Russell Wilder back in the 1920s. An obituary published in the medical journal *Diabetes*[175] credits him as being the first to demonstrate the 'effectiveness of a ketogenic diet in the treatment of epilepsy'.

The use of the ketogenic diet in the management of epilepsy is probably the closest that food comes to being medicine. Before you think I've changed my mind on the use of the phrase 'food is medicine' and the potential harm that using it can do, I haven't. Don't panic.

All ketogenic diets are incredibly high in fat. They tend to work in ratios, with the classic keto diet using a ratio of 4:1, meaning that for every 4 grams of fat there is 1 gram of either protein or carbohydrates. This means that in every meal, 90 per cent of the energy comes from fat, with about 6 per cent from protein and 4 per cent from carbs. Not everyone does it this way though, with the next most common ratio being 3:1. This still results in a whopping 82 per cent of the energy coming from fat.

As we talked about in the last chapter, the Mediterranean diet, commonly regarded as the gold standard when it comes to health and life expectancy, has a split of around 40 per cent fat, 20 per cent protein and 40 per cent carbohydrates. Only slightly different, eh?

So, what's the reason for consuming that much fat? Well, the main purpose is to go into something called ketosis. As we've already covered in the chapter on carbohydrates, the main energy source for the cells in our body is glucose. In situations where we run out, for example during times of starvation, the body has different mechanisms in place in order to stay alive and functioning. One of these is the ability to utilise fat for energy. Fat is converted by the liver into ketone bodies, more commonly known as ketones, which can then be used in place of glucose.

There are actually very low levels of ketones in the blood at all times, seeing as fat turnover never actually stops. Whenever the need for energy increases, and there isn't any glucose around, these levels go up slightly. To be classed as being in ketosis, the ketone levels need to go above 0.5 mmol/l (millimoles per litre), something that will be relevant later on.

The idea behind ketogenic diets is to force the body to increase ketone production throughout the day, as the restriction of carbohydrates means that it's never provided with enough glucose. Protein levels in the diet also have to be kept relatively low as otherwise it can be converted into glucose and slows ketone production.

Now, from a medical perspective I find the fact that this can help in the management of epilepsy absolutely fascinating. There is something about the brain having to use ketones for energy when there's no glucose left that appears to help in what is known as 'refractory epilepsy' – defined as when at least two different antiepileptic drug schedules have failed to provide sustained relief from seizures. The exact reason as to why it has the potential to help though is still unknown, even after a century of research[176].

It's really important to acknowledge that there is only good evidence for the ketogenic diet showing some benefit when medication has failed. In patients where medication has worked, the ketogenic diet is not advisable. It cannot cure epilepsy, nor replace working medication. This is again a reminder as to why the phrase 'food is medicine' is unhelpful. In cases of refractory epilepsy, the success rate of the ketogenic diet to reduce seizures varies wildly and seems to have better outcomes in children[176].

As with all management of medical conditions, if you are living with epilepsy and are tempted to try a strict keto diet yourself, please make sure it's under the supervision of your doctor. Diets that drastically restrict whole macronutrient groups not only have the potential to impact your relationship with food and affect your mental health, but can also lead to nutrient deficiencies if not done properly. This leads to the ketogenic diet being incredibly hard to stick to, with some studies showing a dropout rate of up to 82 per cent[177]. Cutting out lots of food can also lead to an accidental reduction in energy intake, something crucially relevant when it comes to children as it has the potential to result in permanent growth delay[178]. Lastly, one study reported that 10 per cent of children they attempted to treat with the ketogenic diet experienced serious, potentially life-threatening complications, most within a month of starting on it[179].

A strict ketogenic diet is not something to be jumping headfirst into without proper thought. I want to be clear about that.

Becoming a fad diet

Like pretty much everything to do with food it didn't take long before the ketogenic diet got turned into one for weight loss. Are you really that surprised? I was given permission to share the following message that I was sent over social media and I think it sums things up quite succinctly:

'I attempted the keto diet (complete with urine test strips to test for "being in" ketosis) in an attempt to lose weight two years ago. Although I ended up with all the features of typical keto sickness (dizziness, irritation, fatigue, headaches) I still kept going!!!! Idiot. I tried so hard to get enough fibre in because I found that consuming that much fat and protein really, REALLY messes with your gastrointestinal tract. I loved fruit before going keto and cutting it out of my diet made me surprisingly depressed.

Overall, I quit keto after three months because it made me feel sluggish, gave me bowel upset, the power and strength in my lifts was down, was consistently having headaches, when before this I typically only get one if dehydrated. I lost weight, but I also lost feeling myself.'

What tends to convince people that the keto diet is going to work for weight loss is the fact that your body is using fat for energy. At first glance this sounds like a no-brainer, but like everything else with the body it's really not that simple – we'll explain why in a bit. Like all fad diets for weight loss I hope that this one will eventually fall by the wayside, but I've a feeling it's going to take longer than most . . . hence the reason for giving it almost an entire chapter to itself.

Whenever I talk about ketosis on social media, I often get asked if it's the same as diabetic ketoacidosis (DKA). As we've touched on already, DKA is a dangerous situation that can occur in people with diabetes when there's a lack of insulin, such as if missing doses or in times of infection that can counter the insulin that might be present. Without insulin the glucose can't be transported into the cells for energy and there's an uncontrolled production of ketones at an incredibly fast rate in order to make up for this. These ketones make the pH of the blood more acidic at a rate that the body isn't able to manage.

The reason why this is different to deliberately causing ketosis through diet is because of the speed of ketone production. Having no insulin causes very fast ketone production whereas having no glucose causes a more controlled one. There are a couple of case reports of people ending up in ketoacidosis as a result of the keto diet[180,181] but this fortunately appears to be pretty rare.

So why wouldn't weight loss be inevitable if your body is using fat for energy? The thing that trips most people up is that it's not body fat that's being used, but the *dietary fat* being eaten. Weight change is always governed by energy balance. You can't trick your body into reducing levels of body fat unless it has to, otherwise we'd have died out as a species long ago.

When you eat lots of fat and drastically reduce carbohydrates, the body uses the fat you've eaten to form ketones and use as energy. If you don't eat enough food it will use some of your body fat for energy instead. The latter is not unique to a ketogenic diet.

The second thing that trips people up is the fact that weight loss seems to occur really quickly on a ketogenic diet, which tricks people into believing it must be super-effective. As we talked about earlier, excess glucose is stored not only as fat but as glycogen, which is stored in our liver and muscles. When we remove carbohydrates from our diet, the body first uses up its stores of glycogen in order to try to maintain blood glucose levels. Glycogen is actually stored alongside three to four parts water, meaning that when it's broken down the associated water is then excreted in our urine. The initial fast drop on the scales that is often seen with the ketogenic diet is mainly due to the loss of water weight[88].

This also means that when someone introduces carbohydrates back into their diet, weight gain seems to occur even if the person is not in a positive energy balance. This is because, as the body replenishes its stores of glycogen, it has to retain water to do so.

It's a good reminder that weight changes are often as a result of things that have nothing to do with fat.

As we move on to looking at some of the myths and common misconceptions surrounding the ketogenic diet, I want you to hold one question in the back of your mind. When you deprive your body of its main source of energy it finds a way to survive in the form of ketones. Is survival really all you're aiming for?

'THE KETOGENIC DIET IS THE BEST DIET FOR WEIGHT LOSS'

That would be a no (as a reminder, there really is no such thing as the 'best' diet for weight loss – they are all equally as unsustainable as each other). Weight gain is incredibly multifactorial and choice of food intake is only one piece of a massive puzzle.

Now if we *were* to label something the 'best' diet for weight loss it would have to meet a few different criteria:

- It should lead to more weight loss than other diets.
- It should be easier to stick to than other diets (be more sustainable).
- It should be (at the bare minimum) health-promoting.

Trying to assess research studies that use a ketogenic diet is actually incredibly hard. In order for someone to be in ketosis they have to be eating so few carbs (and so little protein) that the level of ketones in their blood reaches *above* 0.5 mmol/l. Any increase in carbohydrate intake leads the body to default back to using glucose for energy and the ketone levels to drop.

A review looking at 62 different studies using a ketogenic diet found that only 25 of them (around 40 per cent) used macronutrient ratios that would have actually led to ketosis[182]. This might sound like semantics, but the whole point of the many ketogenic diets out there is the supposed benefit of the ketones. If not, it's just another low-carb diet, something we've talked about already (see page 90).

Studies that take place on a metabolic ward (where participants live full-time at a research unit and only have access to food that they're specifically given), tend to result in ketosis quite reliably. On the flip side, the studies where people go about their daily life while taking part don't. The ketone levels in about 80 per cent of the latter never go above 0.5 mmol/l[183], meaning that only one in five people manage to stick to the diet well enough to be in ketosis. None of the studies actually acknowledge that as a problem, but I'd argue it gives us some clue as to how hard the ketogenic diet truly is to stick to.

Is the ketogenic diet better for weight loss?

Research would suggest not. In comparison to other diets, it shows that participants might lose *slightly* more weight at 12 months on a ketogenic diet, but this could very much be down to water loss as explained earlier. The higher-quality studies (such as the ones that actually make certain that the participants are in ketosis, among other things) show absolutely no difference in weight loss[184].

Some advocates of the ketogenic diet claim that energy balance doesn't matter when glucose is out of the picture. This is simply not true. There are many, many things that impact energy balance, but in the end if the amount of energy *in* is less than the amount of energy *out*, then weight loss occurs. It makes no difference whether that energy is coming from fat, carbohydrates or protein.

To show that any weight loss that might occur with the ketogenic diet is still entirely governed by energy balance, we can look at a recent study in which participants spent four weeks on a high-carbohydrate diet, followed by four weeks on a ketogenic one[185]. Both diets contained exactly the same amount of energy. Every single thing that the participants did was controlled and measured on a metabolic ward. The result? The researchers found that there was absolutely *no difference* in body fat loss between the two diets. None.

Is it easy to stick to?

The simple fact is that, for most people, the ketogenic diet is really hard to maintain for very long. An analysis of all weight-loss studies over the last decade that looked specifically at adherence found that, on average, you can expect around 60 per cent of people to stick to their chosen diet[186]. Looking at research studies where the ketogenic diet has been given for refractory epilepsy (not weight loss) the adherence sits at around 40 per cent[187]. Add in the fact that only 20 per cent of people are able to stick to the diet well enough to be in ketosis (see above), and I'd argue that this is likely to be closer to the real number.

A reminder that these studies aren't true to the real world. The participants are being brought into a study centre, usually once a week, for body measurements and diet consultation. They are usually given journals and detailed food composition lists. If you take all of that directed support away and picture the average person who's gone on the ketogenic diet because their friend told them to, I'd argue the true adherence rates will be even lower than 20 per cent.

Have you heard of 'the keto flu'? Nausea, headaches, fatigue and sugar cravings are very common in the first couple of weeks. This is as a result of the brain struggling to cope without glucose. It's no wonder that it's not particularly easy to stick to.

Irrespective of what those who promote a ketogenic diet might tell you, there is absolutely zero evidence that it stops weight from being put back on any more than any other diet. That kind of claim is utter nonsense.

Is the ketogenic diet 'healthy'?

The simple answer is no.

The ketogenic diet removes large quantities of micronutrient-rich foods such as vegetables, fruits, legumes and grains. As such, there is a very real risk of becoming nutrient-deficient. There's been research into this that analysed the micronutrient content of an optimal ketogenic diet; one where the most nutrient-dense foods possible were chosen[188]. Even with 'ideal' conditions it still resulted in 19 out of the 24 vitamins and minerals analysed being below the recommended intake. Eleven of them were at less than

50 per cent of what they should have been. This isn't trivial. Real-world analysis would show even worse deficiencies, as it's an incredibly privileged position to be able to choose the most nutrient-dense foods, one that many won't be in.

There's more great news. The ketogenic diet has the real potential to increase cardiovascular risk. It's commonly very high in saturated fat, often double the recommended limit. Research has shown the ketogenic diet increases LDL cholesterol and decreases HDL cholesterol after only six weeks, irrespective of any change in weight[106,189]. This is not something to be glossed over.

Finally, don't forget that we have a relationship with food. From a psychological perspective, diets that drastically restrict food groups or macronutrients are incredibly problematic. They have the potential to increase the risk of disordered eating behaviours including bingeing, obsession with food, anxiety and mood changes.

In conclusion: the ketogenic diet doesn't lead to more sustainable weight loss. It's difficult to maintain due to how restrictive it is, it leads to nutrient deficiencies and carries with it the real risk of cardiovascular disease. There's no best diet for weight loss anyway, but objectively the ketogenic diet would definitely be somewhere near the bottom. If you really enjoy eating that way, I'm not here to stop you. Just please stop misleading others by minimising the real problems with it.

'THE KETOGENIC DIET CAN CURE TYPE 2 DIABETES'

I'm going to talk about type 2 diabetes 'remission' in this chapter and steer clear of the word 'cure'. We tend to do so in the medical world; with type 2 diabetes being so multifactorial (see page 101) it's almost impossible to guarantee that it will never come back.

Food *can* play a part in the management of type 2 diabetes, seeing as anything that reduces blood glucose levels can be beneficial. As discussed already (see page 99), that might include the reduction of carbohydrates[190]. The ketogenic diet is an extreme example of that – by not providing the body with glucose and forcing it to use ketones for energy instead, the average blood glucose levels will come down. For some patients this may even mean that they can come off their anti-diabetic medications. Sounds like remission to me!

Kind of. The problem here is that by removing carbohydrates the underlying insulin resistance is only being masked. It doesn't go away. When carbohydrates are reintroduced the blood glucose levels shoot right back up again. *This is not remission.*

The only thing that has been shown to actually restore pancreatic beta cell function and reverse the insulin resistance (true remission) is weight loss[191]. Can the ketogenic diet lead to weight loss? Sure, but as we've already covered it isn't special in that regard and it certainly isn't any more sustainable than any other fad diet.

It's important to note that weight loss itself isn't a guaranteed fix either. Even in the DiRECT trial[191], widely considered to be the gold standard when it comes to remission through weight loss, there were significant numbers of participants who lost substantial weight but didn't go into remission. This is often related to the duration of diagnosis, with the longer the participants having had type 2 diabetes, the less likely remission being to occur, full stop. The participants started with 12 weeks of drastic energy restriction in the form of soups and shakes, followed by reintroduction of solid food. Like in all weight-loss studies, despite incredibly close support and monitoring, almost all of the participants started to regain weight after that first period, with smaller numbers sustaining remission as weight regain occurred.

So, in conclusion, the ketogenic diet might improve symptoms of diabetes by making glucose control easier, but it isn't special when it comes to true remission. It's not accurate to claim that the ketogenic diet is the cure for type 2 diabetes.

'THERE ARE NO DOWNSIDES TO FOLLOWING A KETO DIET'

With keto having become a bit of a cult in recent years there's been a tendency for those who promote it to claim that literally everyone should be eating that way. 'There are no downsides!' they proclaim. That's simply not true.

We've already talked about the potential health risks, so what I thought I'd do is hand this section over to people who contacted me on social media to share their experiences. It's very easy to stumble across endless praise for the ketogenic diet online, so I think it's important that you have a more balanced picture:

'All I ever hear is good things about keto and it's annoying! I tried it after it was sold to me as a good thing because I have PCOS. Made me feel like absolute shit, didn't make me lose any more weight than just simply being in a calorie deficit, gave me horrendous stomach pains and diarrhoea, and eventually made my skin so dry that parts of my skin just split from touching it. Worst "diet" I've been on. It was also one of the most difficult for me to stick to because being a vegetarian I felt like all I could eat was lettuce, cheese and eggs.'

'I did the keto diet for about 8–10 months, starting about 5 years ago. I was reasonably young (a.k.a. impressionable) and desperate to lose weight because of how I felt viewed by society and even some of my family. I lost weight during that time, but I was absolutely at my most unhealthy, especially mentally. I was miserable on the inside, but because people in my life kept praising my weight loss, I kept chasing to lose more because those comments made me feel of value. I was really strict with myself and what I could eat, even at social gatherings. I would go to family holiday meals and just eat the salad and meat. I would go out to dinner with friends and only order salads off the menu and request them without any of the higher carb things they might come with. If I drank alcohol while socialising, it was only hard liquor mixed with diet soda. All this made me start to dread social events. Along with all of that it also led to massive binges. I would stuff myself full of all the food I had been depriving myself of in the privacy of my bedroom. I would eat so much chocolate/chips/baked goods that I would feel nauseous. I could feel my body being full but I'd just keep going. I'd feel like a monster and the next day I'd be even stricter about what I ate, something which became a vicious cycle. That was five years ago and I'm still unpacking and unlearning aspects related to these habits. I'm still having to put thought every day into being gentle and kind with myself about what I eat. I've had colleagues find out what I used to look like and they've asked how I did it. I tell them it was keto, but I also tell them that I would 100 per cent never do it again and would NEVER suggest that someone else do it.'

'I got told by my GP to go on the keto diet as apparently this was the only way I'd lose weight. He told me I needed to lose weight due to having PCOS (even though my symptoms were minimal). I tried it for six weeks and I passed out four times during that time. I had migraines, body aches, felt faint all the time and had heart palpitations to name but a few things. I told my GP about this and his response was, "but you've lost weight yes?" Safe to say I soon put back on everything I'd lost and more. I have absolutely no support from my GP now due to having "failed".'

'My husband and I tried keto for about 10 days and I felt terrible the whole time. Nauseous every time I worked out and I was stressed about how long it took me to prep my food without my usual carbs. I lost a bit of weight, but it wasn't worth it. The counting and label reading made me more stressed about the food I was eating and I didn't enjoy cooking anymore because I had to eliminate ingredients I liked a lot. One evening, after my husband and I got back from our after-dinner walk I felt so sick. Ended up vomiting four times in the next few hours and I think it had to do with all of the heavy food we'd eaten. That turned me off from it entirely and we went back to eating our normal diet again within a couple days. Keto is something that some people swear by but it wasn't sustainable for us. Mentally and how it made me feel physically were a huge turn off.'

'I'm an endurance athlete. Around four years ago I went super low-carb (I was in ketosis through glycogen depletion from exercise). I bought into the hype about being "fat adapted" and not needing to eat during longer runs as I had suffered from some GI issues. Long story short: amenorrhea, seven stress fractures, osteoporosis, a terrible relationship with food and some pretty awful psychological and physiological issues. I went from running for my country to an injured, depressed mess. This was directly due to low energy and carbohydrate availability. I remember vividly waking up the morning after a race sweating pure ammonia as my body broke down my muscles. It makes me so angry when people push these diets without actually understanding the potential consequences.'

These were just a small selection of the many messages I received. Are there people who really enjoy the keto diet? Sure. Are there people who think that they're enjoying it until it all goes horribly wrong and backfires? Many of the messages I received would corroborate an answer of yes to that as well.

One of the biggest red flags to me is the experience of the 'keto flu' as mentioned earlier. In any normal circumstance things like nausea, headaches and fatigue would be a good sign that maybe you should change what you're doing . . . but the common reply is just to push through and get used to it. It's not logical.

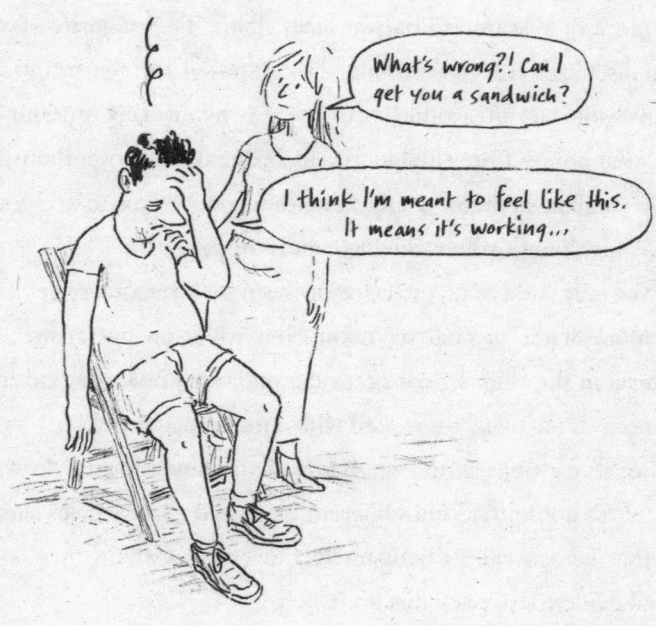

When your body is telling you to stop doing something it's usually best to listen to it.

'KETOSIS CHANGES VAGINAL ODOUR'

Can a keto diet really change the odour of your vagina? It turns out that this is likely to be just another example of society obsessing over what vaginas should smell like. Colloquially termed 'keto crotch', it refers to a supposed change in vaginal odour and irritation after changing to a ketogenic diet. People have theorised that this is as a result of unwanted bacterial growth, secondary to ketones making the pH in the area more acidic.

The thing is, at the time of writing this, I couldn't find even one piece of research to back up this claim. The majority of vaginal discharge is mucus produced by glands of the cervix and sits at an acidic pH of around 4.5. There is a very tiny amount of fluid that comes from the blood vessels directly through the walls of the vagina, so theoretically, ketones might be able to arrive via that route. That's where the logic ends though.

Not only is there no evidence of those on a ketogenic diet having more acidic vaginal secretions, but when an overgrowth of bacteria in the vagina does occur (a condition known as bacterial vaginosis) it's actually associated with a more *alkaline* pH[192].

So, if it's not vaginal secretions, is it something to do with sweat? It's not hard to find different blogs and news articles claiming that ketosis causes bad-smelling sweat, but again there's no actual evidence to back this up.

After ketones are broken down for energy, they produce compounds that have to be got rid of by your body. Some of them come out in your breath (resulting in bad breath that smells a bit like nail varnish remover/pear drops) with the rest being excreted in your urine. Sweat? Not so much.

Are there anecdotal tales of people believing that their vagina smells differently after going on a ketogenic diet? Sure. Might it actually be that they're misinterpreting the altered smell of their own breath? Possibly. Whatever the actual reason, diet being the cause really shouldn't be on the list. If your vagina smells different to normal, the safest thing to do is see a doctor about it.

'THE KETOGENIC DIET CURES MENTAL HEALTH DISORDERS'

This shit makes me mad.

First off, mental health is incredibly multifaceted. Unless a nutritional deficiency is *directly* causing said mental health disorder, food isn't going to cure it. Second, why the hell would keto cure it?! Mental health conditions don't develop because your brain suddenly decides that it no longer wants glucose. Remember, ketones are what your brain lives off when it *has* to, not because it wants to.

People will point towards the potential benefits of a keto diet for refractory epilepsy and claim it must therefore be a good thing for any conditions related to the brain, but that's still not a good argument. Not only is the mechanism by which ketosis sometimes helps in epilepsy unclear, but research looking specifically at mental health doesn't agree with them either.

A systematic review a few years ago wasn't exactly what you'd call encouraging[193]. To start, half of the available studies were in animals, with the few individual case studies and small trials in humans all showing mixed results. The researchers summed it up very politely when they stated that there was: 'insufficient evidence for the use of [the ketogenic diet] in mental disorders, and it is not a recommended treatment option.'

In conclusion, there's no evidence for ketosis curing mental health disorders and it should be immediately challenged whenever claimed. Not only do restrictive diets actually have real potential to *worsen* your relationship with food and mental health, but the insinuation that those who might be struggling simply aren't 'eating correctly' is rhetoric that should never be tolerated.

'KETONE DRINKS CAUSE WEIGHT LOSS'

Every week that goes by at the moment brings with it yet another online advert selling ketone supplements. These are usually in the form of drinks/shots that are sold as an easy method to put your body into ketosis and burn fat.

What a load of crap.

When you drink ketones in liquid form, they cause a transient rise of ketones in the blood after your body absorbs them[194] . . . but what does this achieve? The length of time that you technically go into ketosis for is going to be dependent on how many ketones you consume and whether you have eaten, or are about to eat, food with carbohydrates in it. Your body uses up these ketones for energy and then carries on as normal. It doesn't magically cause fat loss.

If you are eating a ketogenic diet already, then ketone drinks could probably act like an energy drink of sorts, but for everyone else they're pretty pointless. They are stupidly expensive and there's no evidence of them doing anything beneficial for your health. Side note: there's also no evidence that drinking ketones will reduce symptoms of the 'keto flu', despite this often being claimed by the companies that sell them.

Stop wasting your money.

Intermittent fasting or privileged starvation?

The reason why I've put intermittent fasting and the ketogenic diet in the same chapter is because the two are often found being promoted by the same people as both of them involve ketones. When your body goes for a prolonged period without food (fasting), stores of glucose get used up and the body starts to produce ketones for use as energy, similar to when carbohydrates are restricted. Having said that, there are plenty of misconceptions around fasting that have nothing to do with eating copious amounts of fat, so let's try to address some of them, shall we?

Intermittent fasting describes an eating pattern where food is confined to a specific time period. The rest of the time is spent in a fasted state, only consuming water and other drinks such as black coffee or tea. If you've ever had an operation at the hospital, you'll have heard the phrase 'clear fluids' to represent these liquids that don't contain any energy. You might be surprised to hear that we all intermittently fast on a daily basis. Unless you're someone who wakes up in the middle of the night for a snack, the reason the first meal of the day is called 'breakfast' is because it literally breaks the fast that has just taken place overnight.

Before we get on to my reservations about fasting for weight loss, please know that I completely acknowledge that fasting has been around for millennia in the context of different religions such as Judaism, Christianity and Islam. The most obvious of these is the month of fasting known as Ramadan, when the vast majority of Muslims around the world fast from all food and drink between sunrise and sunset.

Personally, I believe that there is a big psychological difference between this and fasting in the pursuit of weight loss and/or supposed health. As such, I'm only going to be talking about the latter two going forwards. Having said that though, if you struggle with eating disorders or disordered eating, please note that fasting can be very harmful to both your physical and mental health, irrespective of the purpose.

Shall we address the title of this section? Intermittent fasting *is* privileged starvation, whether you consider it to be that or not. Choosing not to eat, whether it's in the pursuit of weight loss or 'health', is a privilege. Many people do not have this option and live day-to-day not knowing whether they will be able to afford their next meal. Missing a meal isn't fasting for them; it's forced starvation as they have no other choice. Food poverty is very real and we should be careful not to glorify something that for so many is a painful reality.

Choosing to fast in the pursuit of weight loss, in my opinion, brings with it a lot of problems. There will be people who can do so without negatively impacting their relationship with food, but I'd argue that the vast majority who believe they can do so are unknowingly lying to themselves. Diet culture has a habit of normalising eating disorder behaviours; this is no exception. I'm not sure how much more strongly I can put this other than the fact that starving yourself to lose weight is dangerous. It doesn't matter whether you call it intermittent fasting or any other name. Diet culture is sneaky. It helps us justify our disordered eating by wrapping it up in a blanket of supposed wellness. Don't let it trick you.

In order to address some of the misconceptions around what intermittent fasting is supposed to do, let's define what people usually mean when they say that they intermittently fast. The most common iteration of this is what's known as time-restricted feeding. This involves only eating during a certain number of hours each day. This is often in a ratio of 16:8, meaning that people fast for 16 hours of the day and eat during the other 8 hours. This would mean, for example, only eating between midday and 8pm. Others take it to bigger extremes and follow a ratio of 20:4, only eating during a four-hour window, usually at some point in the afternoon. The second most popular form of this is what's known at the 5:2 diet, where people eat normally for five days of the week and then fast during the remaining two. Most people who do this tend not to fast completely but instead just drastically drop their energy intake on those two days.

Intermittent fasting has risen to popularity more recently, with celebrities and wellness gurus alike proclaiming that it's 'fantastic' and allows them to eat 'whatever they like and not gain weight'. Does that sound like a good place to start addressing some of the nutribollocks?

'INTERMITTENT FASTING ALLOWS YOU TO EAT WHATEVER YOU LIKE AND NOT GAIN WEIGHT'

This is misinformation as its finest.

I remember having to challenge a celebrity (who shall remain nameless) on social media over this point. She was talking to her followers via Instagram and told them that intermittent fasting was so easy because 'during your eating hours you can basically eat whatever you want' and that it was during the fasting periods 'when your body burns the fat – especially the belly fat.'

I challenged what she was saying via direct message, but instead of getting defensive and blocking me like the vast majority do, she not only listened to what I had to say but subsequently informed her followers that she may have been wrong and instructed them to go and follow me instead. It slightly backfired as I wasn't quite ready for the sheer number of questions about intermittent fasting that followed! My main takeaway after it all calmed down was that it was surprising just how many people had believed what she'd said as the truth.

A note on weight loss

Let me remind you before we continue that gaining weight is not something that should be avoided at all costs. Society constantly reinforces this rhetoric on a daily basis, through every medium available, and it requires constant challenging to stay ahead of it. Our weight fluctuates – this is completely normal. If you want your choices in life to be based around health, stop ranking your options based on how much weight they're going to make you lose. Weight loss is not synonymous with health . . . because not all weight gain is unhealthy.

Intermittent fasting isn't magical. Restricting the time period in which someone allows themselves to eat can make it difficult to get enough energy in. Think about how much you normally eat during a typical day and then picture trying to cram all that in during the space of four hours. As such, people will often find that they lose weight, but as soon as they stop intermittently starving themselves, their weight goes back to what it was before.

Some will even find that their weight ends up higher. The body has just been put through a period of inconsistent food intake, so it's now keen to store energy in case something similar happens again. In addition, there is great potential for bingeing when food is allowed normally again. Overconsumption of food after underconsumption of food is very normal from a physiological standpoint;

research has shown fasting to be a strong predictor of both binge eating and bulimic pathology[116]. These behaviours can become more engrained and risk the development of an eating disorder, so if any of this resonates with you please don't ignore it. Remember, all this isn't unique to intermittent fasting but can occur with all methods of energy restriction.

How about the claim that it's during the periods of fasting when your body burns the fat? Fat metabolism is in constant turn-over and is determined by overall energy intake. Once the glucose from the last meal runs out the body has stores in the liver that it can tap into, after which it starts to utilise fat for a brief period of time. Any fat that is used is then replaced the next time you eat.

Research backs this up as well. A year-long trial found that there was no benefit to intermittent fasting specifically when it came to weight loss[195]. There was also no difference in where the fat was lost from. The claim that intermittent fasting preferentially reduces belly fat is laughably based on rodent research – you are not a mouse!

Stop thinking that you can trick your metabolism into doing what you want it to. We are evolutionarily hardwired not to lose weight, as weight loss isn't exactly conducive to survival. Refusing to eat except during a small window in the afternoon won't change that. If you're the kind of person who isn't hungry until midday anyway, meaning you never end up eating in the morning, that's absolutely fine. You don't need to change your habits for the sake of it. However, if you absolutely love breakfast, don't let misinfor-mation about intermittent fasting convince you to ignore your normal hunger cues.

'INTERMITTENT FASTING CAN REVERSE AGEING'

In order to function properly, the cells in our body need to have regular clear-outs. Over time waste material builds up and different components within the cell stop working, both of which have to be removed. The technical term for this process is 'autophagy', a word that means self-eating in Ancient Greek and something that every wellness influencer seems to suddenly be an expert in.

As a result of fasting being shown to promote autophagy, it has been claimed to regenerate the immune system, prevent and fight cancer, slow down ageing . . . and many other things that you can easily find with a quick Google search.

Let's explain why none of these things are true.

One of the functions of autophagy is to help recycle parts of the cell in stress conditions like nutrient starvation[196]. All our cells would prefer to be functioning at 100 per cent, but when the body isn't given enough energy for that to happen, a compromise has to be made. This leads to the available nutrients in some cells being recycled and used elsewhere by ones that need them more at that moment in time.

So yes, not eating for a prolonged period does have the ability to encourage autophagy, but you can think of it a bit like choosing to remortgage your house in order to pay the bills after losing your job. It is not something you would necessarily want to do, but it's a fallback option if you have to.

There is absolutely no good evidence that encouraging auto-phagy in the context of starvation does anything more than just move nutrients around. It certainly doesn't have the ability to reverse ageing or anything else magical. Those telling you to starve yourself for health will often quote studies that supposedly prove their claims . . . except they've all been done in mice and parasitic worms. They might resemble parasitic worms, but you definitely don't. This is not good evidence.

The following quote from a research paper[197] sums it up per-fectly: 'it remains practically impossible to monitor autophagy properly in humans'. As such, those who claim that proof exists are either outright lying or just incredibly confused.

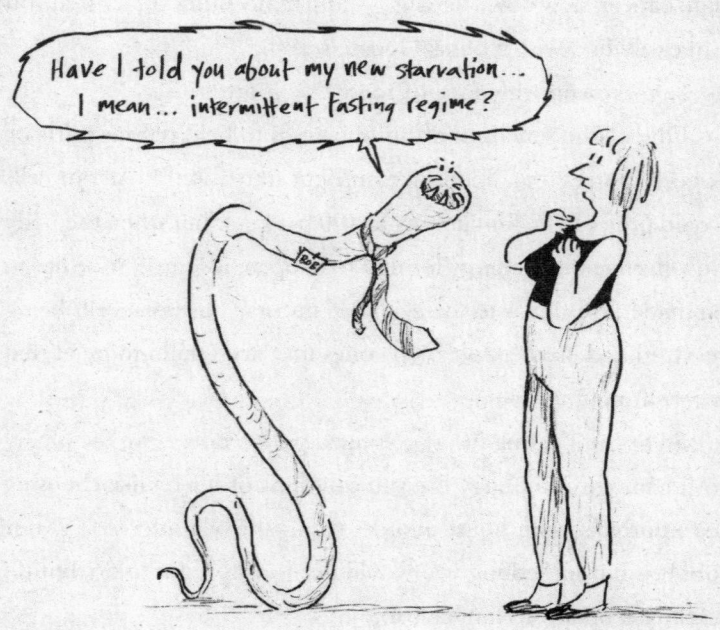

'INTERMITTENT FASTING REVERSES TYPE 2 DIABETES'

I'm going to keep this brief. As we discussed earlier, the only thing that has shown potential in the literature to lead to true remission of type 2 diabetes is weight loss. Can intermittent fasting lead to weight loss in the short term? Sure, starvation will do that. Is there any guarantee or proof that fasting prevents weight from being regained again? Absolutely not. Intermittent fasting isn't any better than any other diet.

The longest trial comparing intermittent fasting to a normal eating pattern found no difference in weight loss or any metabolic markers after a year[195]. Glucose, insulin levels, inflammatory markers, cholesterol . . . all exactly the same as the group who weren't intermittently fasting.

Stop normalising harmful behaviours

I want to end this chapter by being as clear as possible about my thoughts on the ketogenic diet and intermittent fasting. I think I've been pretty blunt already, but just in case. Both are, unfortunately, booming in popularity and I doubt that's likely to slow down anytime soon. While the overwhelming majority of the health claims are clearly nonsense, people are still choosing to follow these fad diets. I'm not denying the fact that one or other of these may fall under a specific way of eating you enjoy and find works with your lifestyle, but that doesn't stop me from pointing out some of the very real potential harm to both your mental and physical health.

Diet culture has a habit of normalising eating disorder behaviours. It takes things that are objectively harmful and repackages them as perfectly valid methods of weight loss. It's been lying to you. Both the excessive restriction of entire food groups and skipping whole meals are bad for your health.

In the context of intentionally trying to manipulate your weight these behaviours are harmful; the question is just how much. Some people are able to come out the other side without noticing much of an impact, whether that's due to an inability to identify it or a level of unpredictable resilience, but for others that couldn't be further from the truth. The development of eating disorders is complex and we can't always predict who will be affected. Don't play with fire, especially when none of the weight-loss promises you're being sold are even true.

7.

MEAT AND TWO VEG

In this chapter we're going to talk a little bit about dietary extremes when it comes to animal products, from the carnivore diet to veganism. Unfortunately, fallacies are prevalent in both, although if it were a competition for false claims, the carnivore diet would win hands down.

Let's start by talking about veganism. I'm on unstable ground already I know but please put the pitchforks down. Let me make it very clear where I'm coming from before we continue so I can hopefully get to standing on something more solid:

- Plants are incredibly healthy for us and we should eat more of them if we can.
- I believe that the vast majority of those who choose to eat a vegan diet are ethically conscious individuals. Having said that . . . it's an unfortunate reality that the loudest voices in the vegan community have started resorting to cult-like ways of convincing people to listen to them.

- Some individuals with eating disorders use the ethical
  aspect of the vegan diet to justify the restriction that
  comes with it. There are many who may benefit from
  eating animal products as part of their eating disorder
  recovery.

I partially blame non-vegans (including myself) for the creation of
the problem. If we had listened to vegans' valid concerns about the
inhumane slaughter of animals (which is pretty undeniable in large-
scale meat production) rather than laughing at them and mocking
their compassion, they probably wouldn't have had to pull in exag-
gerated health claims too . . . like the insistence that going vegan
cures all chronic disease. That's not how food works. It's not medicine remember? As a result of the more militant vegans, there are

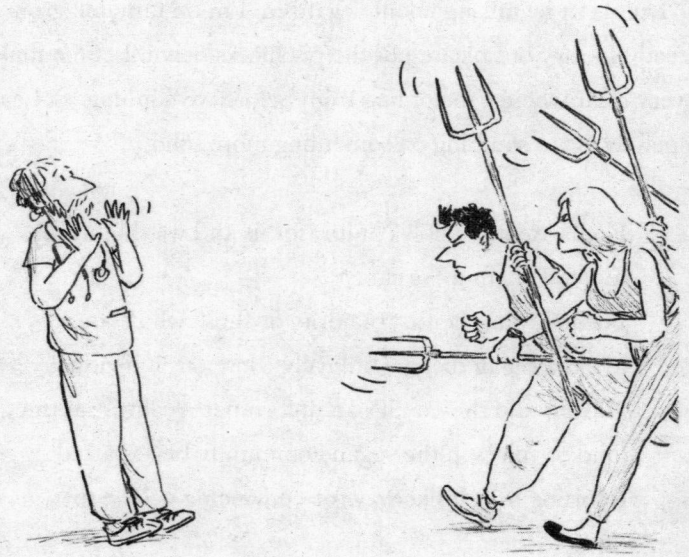

many people who have been put off from realising the health benefits of consuming more vegetables, which is a real shame.

The ethical component of choosing to eat a vegan diet has blurred the lines between choice and belief system. There's a reason why it's called 'veganism'; the -ism at the end of the word implies a doctrine or practice. At the beginning of 2020, a judge in the UK ruled that ethical veganism constitutes a 'philosophical belief' that should be protected by law against discrimination under the UK's Equality Act. This makes it incredibly hard to challenge any misinformation that a vegan might believe as it can feel like a personal attack on who they are. I promise that it's not. I have the utmost respect for vegans who care about animal welfare and encourage people to reduce their meat consumption while also recognising the socio-economic privilege in being able to do so in a Western society. The two *must* go hand in hand.

At the time of writing this there isn't a single vegan 'documentary' that isn't full of cherry-picked evidence and fear-mongering around animal products. I wish that weren't the case, but it is. *The Game Changers*, *What the Health* and *Forks Over Knives* all work from the same rhetoric that eating animal products can't ever be healthy. Nutrition isn't black and white. Belief systems are though.

'VEGAN DIETS ARE ALWAYS HEALTHIER THAN ONES WITH ANIMAL PRODUCTS'

You don't have to look very hard to find people selling you a vegan diet with the promise of health. As much as there doesn't *have* to be anything specifically 'unhealthy' in the choice to only eat plants, that doesn't mean that the opposite is always true.

Let me be clear: you can be perfectly healthy and include animal products in your diet.

Meat can be a great source of complete protein and iron, eggs are crammed with micronutrients and dairy is an important source of calcium for many people. Oily fish is a brilliant source of polyunsaturated fats and can be really beneficial for heart health. It's simply incorrect to pretend that these things aren't true.

You will often hear that a vegan diet is healthier than the typical Western diet, something that is probably closer to the truth. The typical Western diet is often high in red and processed meat, highly processed fried food and refined carbohydrates and low in fresh vegetables. None of which are inherently evil or necessarily unhealthy on their own, but it's not great when they make up the majority of what's being eaten. In that situation, a vegan diet that contains lots of fresh fruit and vegetables, wholegrain carbohydrates, pulses, nuts and seeds is likely going to be more nutritious.

However, a diet that consists of fries, pizza, baked beans and crisps would be considered vegan as well. I'm not sure that many people would argue in favour of that being more nutritious than the typical Western diet. Research has shown that a diet high in what were classed as 'less healthy plant foods' (sweetened beverages, refined grains, fries, sweets) was associated with worse relative cardiovascular risk than a diet including animal foods, with a nutritious omnivorous diet being pretty much identical to one with mainly plants[198].

When comparing dietary patterns, it's important to remember that it's not only diet that impacts our health; the Nurses' Health Study (one of the largest studies looking into chronic disease risk factors in women) showed that meat eaters were more likely to smoke, have a higher alcohol intake and reduced physical activity[199]. Those with these unhealthy lifestyle factors were also more likely to consume less fibre, fruit and vegetables. Very similar characteristics have been shown in cohorts with both sexes[200]. This is all going to have far more of a negative impact on your health than the specific act of consuming meat . . . but that doesn't make for a good headline now does it?

In conclusion, we can encourage people to eat more plants without insisting on demonising animal products, something that I'd argue would actually be far more effective at leading to change.

'MILK CONTAINS PUS'

Have you heard the claim that milk contains millions of pus cells? It's difficult to know exactly how this nutribollocks started, but it is now being propagated by none other than PETA[201]. A page on their website about cow's milk states that: 'white blood cells – also known as "pus" – are produced [in milk] as a means of combating infection.' This is just simply incorrect – white blood cells are not the same thing as pus. Pus is a fluid that mostly consists of bacteria and dead white blood cells. This is not a question of semantics but one of accuracy.

As much as I respect PETA for bringing the issue of animal

cruelty and exploitation out into the open, their track record when it comes to science is shockingly bad. They often use fear-mongering misinformation (also known as lies) about the consumption of animal products in order to make their arguments more persuasive. The ironic thing is that lying to people usually backfires when it comes to convincing them to try a new way of life (in this case going meat-free), so they're probably shooting themselves in the foot.

Seeing as there's no scary-sounding pus in cow's milk, what about the white blood cells then – should we be worried about them? The short answer is no. White blood cells are measured in milk as a marker of safety. If the cow has an infection the number of white blood cells go up and the milk is thrown away. Farmers actually get paid more for lower levels and are penalised (including the risk of having their right to sell milk removed) if the milk repeatedly goes over the limit. This encourages farmers to keep their cows as healthy as possible.

There is no evidence that the presence of white blood cells in milk is a concern to our health, but even if it was, guess what? The process of pasteurisation kills cells, as well as any bacteria that happen to have found their way in. If any white blood cells are left, they would then be killed by the extreme pH of your stomach acid. Facts, not fear.

Pasteurisation is one of the most effective public-health inventions of all time and has made the act of drinking cow's milk incredibly safe. Unpasteurised milk (known as raw milk) carries with it a substantial health risk and is illegal to sell on the high street in the UK. The same laws don't apply in the US, but even

Whole Foods Market over there discontinued selling it due to food safety concerns over a decade ago.

For now, though, let's sum up. There are no pus cells in cow's milk.

'MILK LEACHES CALCIUM FROM YOUR BONES AND CAUSES OSTEOPOROSIS'

Osteoporosis is a condition where a lack of bone density leads to bones becoming weak and brittle over a period of time. Diet can be an important factor, with many different nutrients all playing a role. As a quick run-down: both calcium and phosphate give our bones their strength, with the former accounting for about 30 to 35 per cent of its mass; vitamin D helps us absorb calcium from the gut; and vitamin K helps calcium be deposited in the bones.

Guess what food contains calcium, phosphate and vitamin K? Dairy. Some countries, including the US and Canada, even choose to fortify their milk with vitamin D, making their milk an almost perfect source of all the main nutrients for bone health. With that being the case, it seems pretty weird for milk to have suddenly become public enemy number one, doesn't it?

The main argument on the internet is that the high protein content of dairy makes our blood 'acidic', leading to calcium being pulled from the bones in order to neutralise the acid. This argument is a tiny bit of science mixed with a whole load of wrong. In situations where the pH of our blood does actually become acidic (such as with severe infection, diabetic ketoacidosis or kidney failure) calcium can be lost in the urine[202], but even this doesn't suddenly cause osteoporosis.

Food doesn't have the ability to measurably change your blood pH. If it did, us doctors would have been using it in hospitals across the world for years now! Our blood pH measures between 7.35 and 7.45; when the mechanisms controlling this go wrong, people become seriously unwell and often need admission to ICU. I wish we could give those patients acidic or alkaline diets, but it categorically doesn't work that way.

The breakdown of food *does* generate compounds that are either acid or alkali, but our bodies compensate for the tiny pH changes instantly, treating them essentially as insignificant. Nutrients *can't* act outside of the biological pH range of our blood due to the fact they're not drugs; food isn't medicine.

The protein in milk forms acidic substances after being broken down, but even drinking gallons of the stuff wouldn't do anything significant. It's been shown that protein intake improves calcium retention and bone health[203], meaning this logic is dead in the water many times over.

Dietitians, nutritionists and doctors worldwide are in agreement that dairy is beneficial for our bone health, in both childhood[204] and adulthood[205]. The few rogue quacks you can find on social media aren't a representation of us all, I promise.

If you don't or can't eat dairy for other reasons, make sure you get enough calcium from other food. A large study from the UK found that many vegans had a higher fracture risk due to lower calcium intake[206]. In vegans who were able to consume enough calcium from sources other than dairy this risk disappeared.

'A VEGETARIAN DIET CAN REVERSE HEART DISEASE'

Have you heard of Dr Ornish's Program for Reversing Heart Disease®? It claims that you can reverse heart disease by eating a low-fat, vegetarian diet. It's based on the Lifestyle Heart Trial first published in 1990[207], consisting of 48 patients with coronary artery disease. Twenty-eight were assigned to the experimental group, which included a low-fat vegetarian diet, stopping smoking, stress management training, and moderate exercise, while the other 20 were treated as controls and not asked to make any lifestyle changes.

Coronary artery disease was measured at the beginning of the study and at the one-year mark, by which time the atherosclerotic plaque size had reduced in the experimental group but increased in the control group. Success! There are, unfortunately, many problems with this study from a scientific perspective.

First, this was not solely a dietary intervention. The experimental group exercised and stopped smoking, both of which have good evidence for being beneficial for cardiovascular disease risk[67]. Stress has also been linked with cardiovascular disease risk[208]. Might the low-fat vegetarian diet have been the reason for the reduction in atherosclerotic plaque size? Possibly, but without removing the other variables it's simply incorrect to use words like 'proven'.

Second, and perhaps most damning, is the methodology used to measure atherosclerotic plaque size. Something called quantitative coronary angiography (QCA) was used; a test that has now been superseded due to its limitations[209] by newer tests such as intravascular ultrasound and coronary CT angiography. It doesn't actually measure plaque, but instead measures the diameter of the inside of the artery. That doesn't mean it's useless, but due to its inaccuracy it's been shown that in order to be able to tell if atherosclerotic plaque size is actually changing, a minimum of 0.4mm change in diameter has to be recorded[210]. The Lifestyle Heart Trial doesn't meet this criterion.

In conclusion, not only is it impossible to separate the effects of the other lifestyle interventions from the diet, but we also have no idea whether atherosclerotic plaque size actually changed in the participants due to inaccurate testing protocols. Does this study 'prove' that Dr Ornish's Program for Reversing Heart Disease® works? Absolutely not.

Now you might be wondering why this matters. The issue is twofold. First, Ornish uses his trial as an argument to promote a very low-fat plant-based diet that doesn't allow olive oil. We have evidence that suggests a reduced-fat diet is inferior in comparison to one including olive oil when it comes to cardiovascular events[174], as well as a consensus opinion that extra virgin olive oil is objectively the healthiest source of fat[170]. Second, in 2010, Medicare (the national health insurance programme in the US) decided to cover Ornish's programme. American taxpayers' money is now being spent on something that is based on flawed evidence. From a medical ethics perspective that's a problem.

Is Ornish's programme objectively better than the standard Western diet when it comes to nutrition? Probably. Would it be more ethical to use taxpayers' money to fund a programme that had robust evidence behind it, such as the DASH diet or the Mediterranean diet, instead of one based on a flawed study? I'll let you come to your own conclusion about that one.

'BROCCOLI HAS MORE PROTEIN THAN STEAK'

This claim is often used in response to people saying that you can't get enough protein from a vegan diet. There are actually plenty of sources of protein that aren't animal based, such as seitan, tempeh, tofu, lentils and chickpeas . . . the list goes on.

What confuses me is that instead of picking something like seitan that actually has way more protein per 100g than any steak does, they went with broccoli, which has eight times *less* than steak by weight. It's just completely unnecessary misinformation.

In order to get the same amount of protein from an average 250g steak you would have to eat over 2kg of broccoli. Please tell me you see how ridiculous this comparison is?

There are plenty of reasons to encourage people to eat more vegetables. You don't need to resort to nonsense like this. I know it must be frustrating to have people tell you that you can't get protein from a vegan diet, but two wrongs don't make a right.

'RAW VEGAN DIETS ARE THE HEALTHIEST'

Orthorexia is defined as having an unhealthy obsession with healthy food. The raw vegan diet is a perfect example of that.

People who eat raw vegan refuse to cook any of their food out of fear that the heat will destroy nutrients and make it 'toxic'. They claim by eating everything raw you can cure headaches, allergies, boost immunity and cure chronic disease. It's the same old nonsense. While it's true that boiling vegetables to death can lead to some of the nutrients being left in the water of the pan, normal cooking actually tends to improve digestion and increase nutrient absorption. The slight loss of certain nutrients through cooking is more than made up by the improved digestibility.

Some of the worst misinformation about this comes from vegan blogger Freelee the Banana Girl, who has claimed that a raw vegan diet can fix heavy periods. She is of the unscientific opinion that 'menstruation is toxicity leaving the body' and claims that raw vegan food causes less toxicity and therefore lighter periods.

The truth is actually far more concerning. Research has shown that women on a raw food diet can become so malnourished that around 30 per cent (under the age of 45 years) have partial to complete amenorrhoea (lack of periods). Essentially, they don't have enough body fat for their hormones to function properly and they stop menstruating.

This is not something to be aiming for. Ever.

The discovery of fire and our ability to cook food was a pivotal step in human evolution. Let's not go backwards.

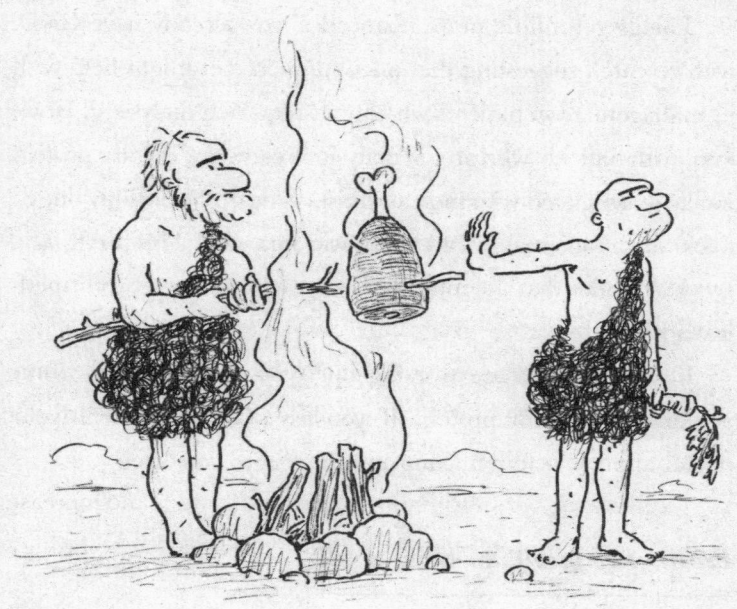

'EATING TOO MUCH PROTEIN CAUSES KIDNEY DISEASE'

This myth has been around for quite a while now. When protein is metabolised by the body, no matter whether it's from an animal or plant source, it ends up eventually producing something called urea, which is then excreted by the kidneys.

The theory goes that by eating too much protein you can overwhelm and damage the kidneys, causing chronic kidney disease (CKD). Research has shown this simply not to be true. If you have healthy kidneys a high-protein diet has absolutely no impact on their function[211].

Things get a little more nuanced if you already have CKD, with research suggesting that a low-protein diet might help with its management in patients who aren't requiring dialysis[212]. However, with patients who are on dialysis already, low dietary protein intake is associated with increased risk of death[213], possibly due to a loss of muscle mass. Told you it was nuanced! This serves as a good reminder that the internet is not the place to get your medical advice.

If your kidneys are working fine, you don't need to worry about eating lots of protein. If you have CKD, talk with your doctor about it before making any changes to your diet.

From only plants to none at all

In recent years there has been a surge of people going to the complete opposite to veganism and following a meat-heavy or meat-only diet. There are some variations, with some adding in eggs, dairy and fish, but there is one constant theme with all of them. Absolutely no plants . . . because plants are apparently toxic.

Unless you're eating something like deadly nightshade (the clue is in the name), this is just nonsense.

There is one fact that pretty much every respected nutritionist, dietitian and medical doctor across the globe agrees on: *plants are incredibly healthy for us and should make up the majority of our diet.* The carnivore diet, as it's named, laughs in the face of this and claims the exact opposite. Not only that, but it's infiltrated the growing toxic masculinity side of wellness culture.

Men, in general, are less engaged when it comes to their medical care and health. They are 24 per cent less likely than women to have visited a doctor within the last year, but are more likely to be hospitalised for preventable illnesses[214]. While it is difficult to pinpoint the exact reasons for these differences, there's certainly a reality to the 'rugged man' stereotype who believes it's weakness to ask for help or care about unimportant things like 'nutrition' (unless of course it's about building muscle).

As a result, most wellness culture has usually chosen to target women as they're more likely to focus on their health and be open to outside influence, resulting in companies like Goop having found their niche. It only takes a cursory look on their website to be able to find vaginal jade eggs claiming to harness 'crystal healing', despite Goop paying $145,000 in settlement in 2017 for making 'unsupported medical claims'[215] in relation to the same product. The only thing a porous jade egg does is increase your risk of dangerous bacterial infections[216].

There have, however, been a few different things that have managed to target men by rebranding themselves as something 'cool' like biohacking, but nothing has played off toxic masculinity quite like the idea of only eating meat. Eat meat, build muscle . . . be a real man. We only have to look at the few identifiable medical doctors who promote the carnivore diet to their followers on social media; each and every one of them has directly encouraged toxic masculinity as a way of promoting their brand. They all spend a decent amount of time lifting weights and have posted photos of themselves shirtless next to ones of vegan doctors who don't have as much muscle, asking their followers who they'd rather look like. When qualified medical doctors are stooping so low as to body shame their colleagues in a plea to promote their fad diets . . . and it's actually working . . . we've got shit to sort out.

'THE CARNIVORE DIET CURES AUTOIMMUNE DISEASE'

There is absolutely no evidence that by removing plants and only eating meat you can cure an autoimmune disease. You might be wondering, therefore, why you can find lots of stories on social media from people who say that you can.

This is all to do with the effects of placebo and confirmation bias. If I give you a tablet and tell you it's going to help when it comes to your health, there is a high probability that it will, even if what I gave you is just made out of chalk. You don't have to be in the dark about it either; research has shown that even when you tell somebody that they're receiving a placebo their symptoms still improve, just not as much as with the real drug[217]. This 'placebo effect' works with any intervention, including both introducing and removing things from someone's diet. As such, it is a really crucial concept to understand in order to challenge some of the 'food is medicine' rhetoric.

The placebo effect is also amplified by 'confirmation bias'. This is the tendency to look for and interpret information in a way that confirms a specific viewpoint. When someone with an auto-immune disease removes plants from their diet, it's because they think it will make them better. Not only will the placebo effect *actually* make them feel better for a while, but they will also subconsciously look for other things to confirm that it has worked. They will link previous meals that included plants with times when their autoimmune disease had been particularly bad, even if there was no real relationship between the two.

What's worse is that if they try to introduce plants back into their diet, the fact that these beliefs are now engrained will actually lead to the placebo effect working the other way round, leading them to feel unwell. This leaves them with only one option – become even more restrictive with what they allow themselves to eat. It can be an incredibly harmful spiral. This is why it's *so* important for a professional (ideally a dietitian or nutritionist) to cast a sceptical eye over what someone believes to be happening.

You may be wondering why all this matters; if people's symptoms are improving surely that's a good thing overall? It matters when the intervention is potentially dangerous or harmful. All restrictive diets carry risk to your mental and physical health, but a carnivore diet is one step above that. Here are just a select few of the reasons why:

- Removing fibre from your diet increases the risk of colon cancer.
- Increasing saturated fat intake increases cardiovascular disease risk.
- Removing all fruit and vegetables increases the risk of vitamin and other micronutrient deficiencies.

One of the most prominent carnivore medical doctors who talks about curing autoimmune diseases with meat, Paul Saladino, admitted recently that he'd been including vast amounts of honey in his diet and had 'immediately felt better'[218]. He tried to brush it off by saying it was due to the electrolytes he was getting from the honey, but that's scientifically nonsense (the amount of stuff other than sugar in honey is next to nothing). It made him feel better because his brain had been craving something other than meat . . . like carbs! He also now admits to regularly eating white rice[219] only nine months after writing a book claiming that these processed carbohydrates were 'universally detrimental' for health[220]. You literally couldn't make this stuff up.

Don't risk your health with nonsense that flies against everything we know to be true about nutrition. The fact that the loudest voices can't even follow their own advice should tell you all you need to know.

'THE CARNIVORE DIET CURES DEPRESSION AND MENTAL HEALTH DISORDERS'

Let's be incredibly clear right from the start. There is absolutely no scientific evidence that by removing all plants from your diet and eating only meat you will be able cure depression or any other mental health disorder. There are a few anecdotal stories of people who claim to have been 'healed' from doing so, but even these are so genuinely concerning to anyone on the outside that I think it's important we go through one of them.

Mikhaila Peterson is a Canadian blogger and wellness guru who sells her own form of the carnivore diet, with her Twitter bio[221] at time of writing stating that her 'autoimmune and mood disorder [is] cured.' Her website describes her background as having been diagnosed with severe juvenile rheumatoid arthritis (an autoimmune disease) at the age of seven and being put on strong immunosuppressant medication at the time[222]. It was so bad that she ended up having both a hip and ankle replacement at the age of 17. She was also diagnosed with severe depression at the age of 12 and 'experienced hypomanic episodes (bipolar type II)' for which she was given anti-depressants. She writes that: 'it finally occurred to me that whatever was happening was likely going to end in my death, and rather soon. After almost 20 years, the medical community still had no answers for me . . . after years of desperate research, I started experimenting with my diet.'

It hurts to read that stuff as a doctor, it really does. As medical professionals we should be paying really close attention to stories like these. Far too many patients with chronic conditions report feeling like the medical community has failed them – we need to be doing better. I'm certainly not here to invalidate her very real experiences in that regard.

Mikhaila went on a self-imposed elimination diet, which she reports cured all of her arthritis and depression within three months. This is, unfortunately, where things start getting problematic. She came off all of her medications, but after becoming pregnant the following year all of her symptoms came back, despite her diet not changing. As is common in these situations, she saw this as a prompt to make her diet even more restrictive, but it didn't resolve her symptoms this time.

Still looking for a solution, she heard about the carnivore diet through an American orthopaedic surgeon called Shawn Baker who happened to be on Joe Rogan's podcast back in 2017. After hearing Baker professing the supposed benefits of eating only meat, Mikhaila decided she would do the same and seemingly hasn't looked back . . . despite experiencing diarrhoea for a month and a half at the beginning. She now claims to be completely symptom-free.

It's at this point I need to introduce you to someone you may have come across already; her father, Jordan Peterson. He's a psychology professor who claims that 'the masculine spirit is under assault' and white privilege isn't real[223], among other things. Toxic masculinity really seems to follow the carnivore diet doesn't it?

This is where it starts to get really weird. Buckle in.

On his own appearance on Joe Rogan's podcast in July 2018, Jordan reports being convinced to go on the carnivore diet after observing his daughter's experience with it[224]. He said that his lifelong depression and anxiety (among a whole host of other things he reported to be suffering with) also resolved and he'd stopped taking his anti-depressants. It wasn't all peachy though. Jordan recounts:

'One of the things that both Mikhaila and I noticed was that when we restricted our diet . . . the reaction to eating what we weren't supposed to was absolutely catastrophic . . . the worst response [was after] we had some apple cider [vinegar] that had sulphites in it . . . it took me out for a month. It was awful . . . It produced

an overwhelming sense of impending doom. I seriously
mean overwhelming . . . I didn't sleep at all for 25 days.'

Jordan was prescribed a benzodiazepine as a result of ongoing anxiety stemming from what he described above. This drug has the
potential to result in severe addiction, something that he noticed
after experiencing withdrawal symptoms two years later when trying to come off it. After multiple failed rehab attempts, he enrolled
in an alternative treatment programme in Russia, where he ended
up being put into an induced coma for eight days after getting
pneumonia. I'm not making this stuff up; all of this information is
readily available online and in different interviews and podcasts.

Throughout this entire period Mikhaila was selling member-
ships to a carnivore diet support club on her website and telling
people that it would not only help them lose weight but cure them
of autoimmune diseases and mental health problems.

This whole story is incredibly concerning to me. As much as I
don't particularly like what Jordan Peterson promotes, I have
absolutely no desire to see people get hurt as a consequence of
dietary misinformation. I'm glad to see that he now seems to be
well and no longer in hospital.

I wanted to have this story documented as a warning to those
who might feel like they're being sucked in by promises similar to the
ones that the carnivore diet makes. Here are some things I know to
be true to allow you to make up your mind about the whole thing:

1. Mental health disorders are neither caused by eating
    vegetables, nor cured by only eating meat.

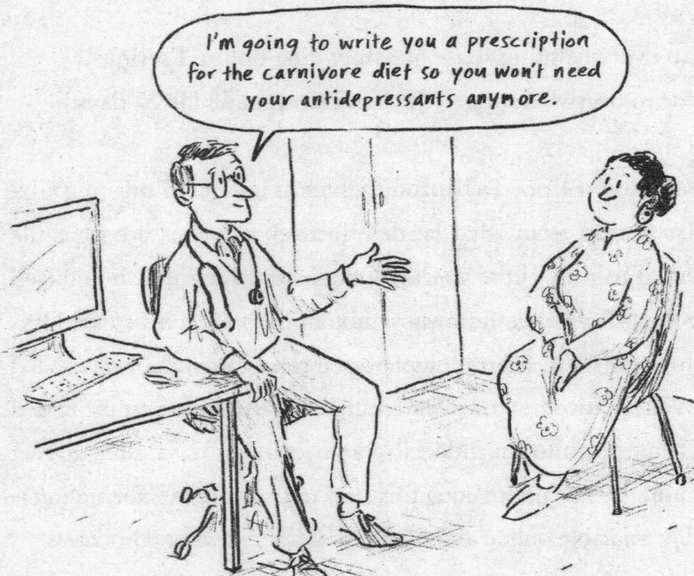

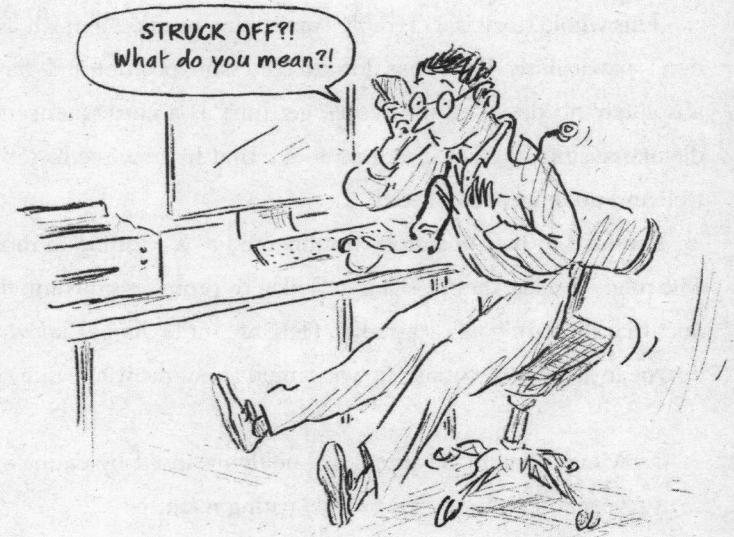

2. It is possible for people to experience an allergic reaction to sulphites in food such as vinegars. What was described by Jordan Peterson, however, doesn't fit the experience of an allergic reaction.

3. A major depressive episode can be characterised by feelings of hopelessness, worthlessness, anxiety and insomnia that can last for over two weeks. This can occur in individuals with depression due to many different reasons, including as a result of coming off therapeutic anti-depressant medications[225].

4. Medication for mental health disorders, while not always needed, can save lives. Taking medication should never be seen as a failing.

5. We need to be better at talking about, and normalising, mental health disorders in order to remove the ongoing stigma that surrounds them. This stigma can often prevent people from seeking help when things go wrong.

Do I think that the people promoting these diets are *deliberately* trying to mislead people? Usually not. Do we still need to challenge it so that other people don't potentially come to real harm? Without a shadow of a doubt.

Eat more plants

Let's not waste any more time on the ridiculousness that is the carnivore diet and instead just reiterate a simple truth:

Plants are incredibly good for your health and you should really be eating more of them.

Aiming to be plant-based (simply meaning 'based around plants') doesn't mean we have to remove animal products in their entirety, but they should certainly step aside and make room for more plants to take up pride of place on our plate.

A final thought to leave you with. It's important to acknowledge with this conversation that depending on the country and area in which someone lives, socio-economics can greatly impact someone's ability to include more plants in their diet. Remember, it's not just about money; time, energy and access to appliances are just a few things that play a role. Buying frozen rather than fresh vegetables is often a cheaper (while equally nutritious) way of getting more vegetables into your diet, but it's useless if you don't own a freezer. Let's make an effort not to unintentionally belittle the situation others find themselves in when we are discussing this stuff. It's far too common to see influencers on social media boiling down the act of improving diet to whether someone 'can be bothered or not'; an opinion that often couldn't be further from the truth. Caveats and nuance are both free and show understanding and compassion.

8.

FOOD CANNOT CURE CANCER

Cancer is a *big* word and one that carries with it quite a lot of emotion and anxiety. It is also something where, despite treatment options improving, we as doctors are often limited with what we are able to do. The medical treatments that are proven to increase survival rates can often have horrible side effects; chemotherapy can make you tired, lethargic and nauseated, hair can be lost and it can put you at higher risk of infections while on the treatment. Radiotherapy carries with it the risk of local complications, skin reactions and even potential secondary cancer years later.

Without an understanding of how cancer develops and why we recommend the treatments we do, it's easy for charlatans to a) convince people that you're responsible for your own diagnosis and b) sell you their snake oil. They offer 'solutions' that don't have any of the nasty side effects the drugs us Big Pharma doctors have been prescribing you – fasting, alkaline diets, cutting out sugar, juicing . . . does any of that sound familiar?

Now, if you've fallen for any of that stuff in the past, or are considering it at present, I'm not here to tell you off or call you stupid.

Instead, let me empower you with knowledge so that not only are you able to recognise the crap but you can also help others avoid a similar fate.

What is cancer?

We have around 37 trillion cells in our body, each of them with a finite lifespan. That's a ridiculous number, so to put it into context, that's about 100 times more than the number of stars in the Milky Way. Yeah, exactly. Every second of every day over 100,000 ageing cells are replaced through the processes of cell division and programmed cell death, both of which are crucial to make sure that our body stays functioning like it should do. One part of this is ensuring that all 6 billion base pairs of DNA are copied correctly, otherwise the new cell won't work properly.

Therefore, with our body having to make 600 trillion new base pairs of DNA every second, it's not too surprising that mistakes are made . . . but they happen more frequently than you'd probably guess; up to 120,000 mistakes every time a cell divides[226]. Thankfully there are multiple checks in place to identify and repair these errors both during and after cell replication. The few that make it through all this and end up becoming permanent are then known as mutations.

The vast majority of mutations don't cause too much of a problem by themselves, but when they build up in genes that manage cell division, programmed cell death and the DNA repair mechanisms just mentioned, they have the potential to result in uncontrolled cell replication and growth . . . also known as cancer.

There are many factors at play when it comes to someone's risk of developing cancer: genetics through inherited mutations, environmental exposure to carcinogens (substances/radiation that increase risk of mutations, often by causing DNA damage) and the simple act of getting older. It often takes multiple different mutations over the course of a lifetime to result in cancer formation; the longer we live the more chance we have of this happening.

The good news is that cancer survival rates have been improving dramatically due to breakthroughs in treatment and earlier diagnosis. In the UK alone cancer survival has doubled over the last 40 years[227]. The bad news is that as time's gone on it's become one of the worst areas for the 'food is medicine' rhetoric to rear its ugly head. Let me say this right at the beginning: *food cannot cure cancer*[228]. There is no nuance here.

Nutrition can *support* a patient through treatment and recovery, but it's less about dietary specifics and more about making sure that enough energy is obtained. Cancer results in the body being in a state where molecules are constantly being broken down in order to produce energy. This includes both fat and muscle. Due to this, weight loss is incredibly common and often one of the first signs that something's wrong. When you add on the fact that cancer treatment can not only leave people nauseated (as mentioned earlier) but also change taste and bowel habit, you begin to understand why the simple task of getting in enough energy can be a problem. Advising someone with cancer to follow the newest fad diet is not only completely pointless but incredibly short-sighted.

We know and accept that people's use of complementary and alternative medicine increases greatly after a cancer diagnosis[229]. It's difficult to know exactly the reasons why, but they can include: liking the idea of a 'natural' or 'non-toxic' option; feeling more in control over decisions about care; and being promised a cure when doctors have labelled something as terminal. Now don't get me wrong; I'm not personally against the use of alternative approaches in a complementary fashion, but as much as these options might help people's symptoms, none of them can actually treat cancer. Unfortunately, they are rarely sold with that much transparency and can lead to people making the heart-breaking decision to choose them *over* conventional treatment.

Research has shown that when patients choose alternative medicine as their only anti-cancer treatment things don't end well[230]. Actually, you know what, let me be clearer than that and not beat around the bush. People die. Women with breast cancer have a more than fivefold increased risk of death. Colorectal cancer – more than a fourfold increased risk of death. Lung cancer – more than a twofold increased risk of death. Even if patients only delay the start of conventional treatment in order to give alternative medicine the old college-try this can greatly worsen survival rates[231].

Cancer nutribollocks isn't a joke and *must* be challenged.

'YOU'VE GOT CANCER BECAUSE [INSERT REASON HERE]'

Every week we're told there's a new reason why we get cancer and the fear-mongering starts all over again. Coffee, shampoo,

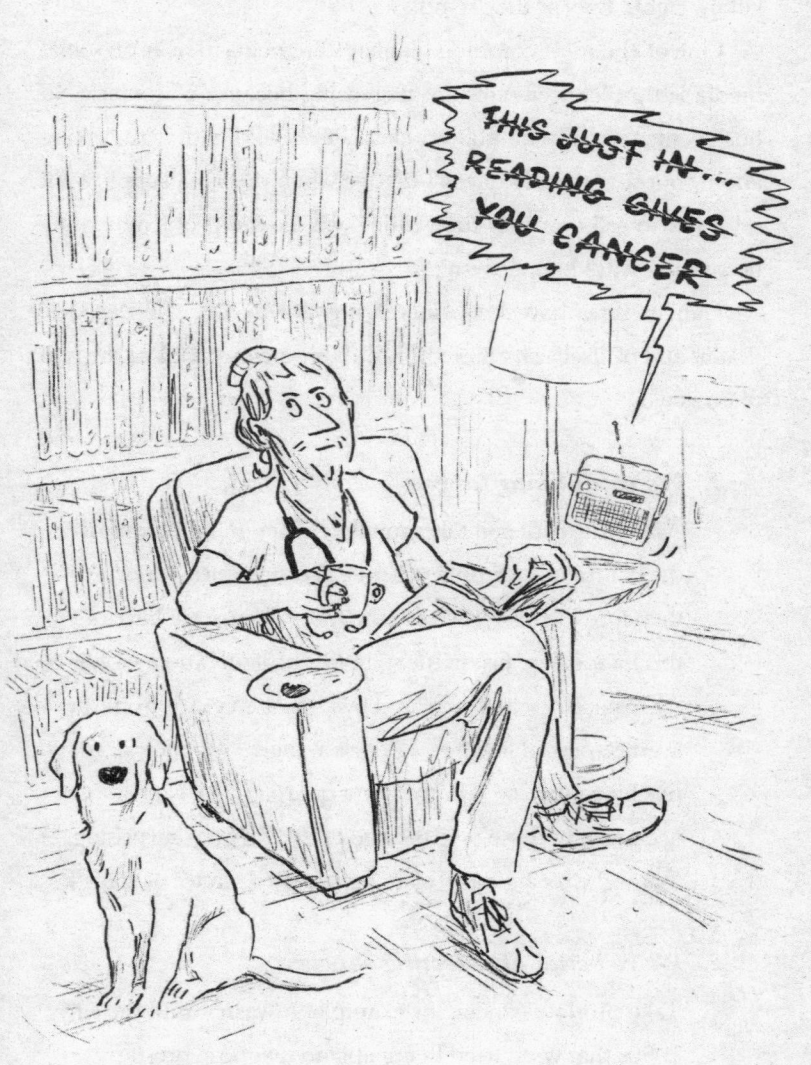

deodorant, plastic water bottles, face masks . . . they're all out to kill us, right? Except they're not.

One of the most common blanket statements to hear on social media is that 'cancer rates are increasing because of toxins'. No one seems to really be able to clarify *what* toxins they're talking about, but that usually doesn't matter when there's a supplement or detox to sell you that they claim will fix the problem. Funny how that always happens isn't it?

Cancer rates have been increasing slowly over the decades; that in and of itself isn't a myth. Let's have a closer look at the real reasons why:

1. *We're all living longer*

   As I wrote earlier, it takes multiple different mutations over the course of a lifetime to result in cancer formation, therefore the longer we live the more chance we have of this happening. Just in the span of one generation, global life expectancy has increased by almost 25 years, from the average person living to 47 back in the 1950s but nowadays reaching over 70[232]. With over a quarter of all cancer occurring in those over the age of 70[233] it's not surprising that we're seeing more of it; it's simply a matter of statistics.

2. *We're better at detecting cancer*

   Take prostate cancer, for example. It wasn't until the early 1990s that we started being able to diagnose prostate cancer using a simple blood test[234], leading to much higher detection rates than before. With the average prostate cancer patient having a five-year survival rate of nearly 100 per cent and a 15-year survival rate of 95 per cent[235], many men will die *with* prostate cancer but not as a result of it. If someone were to just look at the numbers, they might conclude that prostate cancer rates have exploded in the last 30 years, when in fact we've just got much better at detecting it.

Does our lifestyle get off completely scot-free? Of course not, but again, that's not straightforward. The issue often boils down a lack of understanding of the complexity of cancer by the people responsible for spreading the misinformation. For example, people read about chemicals called parabens in cosmetics, find some research that says parabens have been found in breast cancer tissue, and start telling anyone who will listen that shampoo can cause cancer. Cue the creation of a 'paraben-free' shampoo and voilà; people profit off the fear of the misinformed.

Parabens in cosmetics are used to stop the harmful growth of microbes. They are often demonised for supposedly carrying a cancer risk, something that is completely untrue. This hasn't stopped the explosion of paraben-free alternatives. The problem is that the alternatives don't work as well, so you have a much higher risk of using contaminated products and they're also more likely to cause allergic reactions. Not only are there no 'good alternatives' to parabens but they're completely unnecessary!

You have probably heard that the estimated likelihood of being diagnosed with cancer during one's lifetime in the UK now sits at just under 50 per cent[236]. This can feel like a scary statistic, so let's try to look at the positives here: in the UK, survival rates have doubled over the last 40 years. Lung cancer incidence is falling globally after successful public health campaigns to stop people smoking. Death rates from breast, colon and stomach cancer have all declined[233].

Please feel safe in your knowledge that there simply isn't one reason that can be attributed to overall cancer rates; try to keep an eye out for the real agenda behind the claims.

'OB*SITY CAUSES CANCER'

This topic often sparks a lot of emotion, and rightly so. Too often the conversation around weight and cancer risk is used to justify stigma and discrimination. Let me explain what I mean.

Back in 2018, Cancer Research UK (CRUK) released their first 'ob*sity is a cause of cancer' campaign. In the campaign video they asked unsuspecting members of the public to guess what the biggest preventable cause of cancer was after smoking, while handing out fake cigarette packets filled with fries. The billboards carried the same message but without the cigarette packet imagery.

The following year they doubled down and made the billboards look like cigarette packets as well, with the message 'ob*sity is a cause of cancer too'. Smoking and ob*sity are *fundamentally* different. Smoking is a behaviour (albeit one also influenced by socio-economics) and the association of the two fuels the rhetoric that weight gain is a lifestyle choice. It's not. Weight gain isn't a habit to be kicked. Weight gain doesn't risk the health of those around you like smoking can, either.

The chief executive of CRUK said that the campaign goal was 'not to compare tobacco with food'. But that's exactly what it did. The campaign used nonsense sweeping statements like, 'if a person is overweight, they are more likely to get cancer than if they are a healthy weight'[237]. As we've already discussed, a 'high' BMI is close to useless at an individual level (see page 47). A BMI value of 27 would officially put someone in the 'overweight' category, yet a recent study found the BMI associated with the lowest risk of death to be . . . drum roll . . . 27[238]. When a prominent charity with an income of over half a billion pounds each year chooses to ignore the stigma that their public health messaging encourages, it's clear we have more work to do.

When I talked about the campaign on my social media account at the time, I had hundreds of messages from people expressing the abuse and discrimination that they had experienced as a direct result. I still have one of those messages saved on my phone to this day:

> 'Another child at my daughter's sports day actually taunted
> her with the words, "Your mum is gonna get cancer and
> die 'cause she's a fat f*ck" . . . I now have a terrified 10-
> year-old and I feel like I can't show my face at school again
> because I'm so worthless and causing her upset.'

At some point the intention behind the messaging becomes irrelevant and it's the actual outcome that matters. The heartbreaking story above shows just how important it is to be incredibly deliberate about how this topic is discussed; without a true understanding of the multifactorial nature of weight gain it's all too easy to turn this into a discriminatory blame game. With recent estimates suggesting that the prevalence of weight stigma is comparable to rates of race discrimination[239], it's an important variable that has to be considered when looking at associations.

So, where has the idea that 'ob*sity causes cancer' come from? Research has shown there to be an association between larger body weight and cancer risk, but for the *vast majority* of cancers it has not been proven to be the cause. It is incredibly important, therefore, that we look at whether there are other reasons as to why an association exists between body weight and cancer before making the statement that it 'causes it'. Without the lens of weight stigma, we don't have to look very hard to find them.

Of the 11 different cancers associated with increasing body size[240], let's look specifically at oesophageal cancer to see what happens when we remove the lens of anti-weight bias.

The biggest risk factors shown to cause oesophageal cancer are: gastro-oesophageal reflux disease (GORD), smoking and alcohol intake, with all three of these having a common factor – stress. Stress has been shown to be associated with an increased occurrence of GORD and its severity[241,242]; onset of smoking at a young age[243], difficulty with smoking cessation[244]; and increased alcohol use[245].

How might weight stigma impact the association found between increasing BMI and oesophageal cancer? Well, weight stigma is linked to anxiety, depression and higher levels of stress hormones[246]. It's entirely plausible that this increased stress is the true reason for the association rather than the weight itself, yet none of the oesophageal cancer research acknowledges or includes this in the analysis.

This is a problem.

Furthermore, with ob*sity prevalence being highest amongst the most deprived areas of the UK[247], could someone's socio-economic status be yet another variable at play here? Absolutely. We know that poverty creates a context of increased stress[248] just like weight stigma. We know that living in poverty is associated with a reduced intake of fruit and vegetables, something else that has also been shown to increase the risk of developing oesophageal cancer[249].

If you look on the CRUK website they overconfidently state that 27 per cent of oesophageal cancer cases are 'caused' by being overweight and ob*se. The paper that they reference to try to prove this specific claim[250] actually makes it very clear that this association is partly due to the fact that there are simply lots of people in those BMI categories (more people = more cases), while also highlighting the impact that socio-economics has on the data.

It angers me that an ignorance of the impact weight stigma has on health, mixed with an unwillingness to acknowledge factors like poverty, leads to statements that further discriminate whole swathes of the population.

We could take each of the other ten different cancers associated with increasing body size and look at them in the same way as I've done above, but that would require an entire book by itself. Briefly though, even something like breast cancer risk that has a more convincing link with weight isn't entirely straightforward. If the distribution of fat tissue means it's producing oestrogen it then has the potential to increase risk in post-menopausal women, but in pre-menopausal women a higher BMI is actually associated with a *reduced* risk[251]. These nuances are too often completely left out from the conversation, leaving fat patients feeling an over-whelming sense of personal responsibility if a diagnosis occurs.

Stigmatising people under the guise of science is *always* un-acceptable. It leads to those at a higher body weight being ignored and mistreated in clinical settings[252] and believing that their doc-tor would prefer not to treat them[253], both of which lead to avoidance of healthcare altogether[46]. It has to stop.

'SUGAR CAUSES CANCER'

Pretty much the only argument for this is that sugar causes ob*sity, which in turn causes cancer. We've covered both of these in this book already; neither of them are accurate. Section done then?

Just about. If you'll humour me, I'd like to specifically (but briefly) cover the association between sugar-sweetened beverages (SSBs) and cancer, seeing as this tends to be the most commonly used area of research to try to argue the point.

A systematic review in 2017 assessed 13 different studies look-ing at SSBs and cancer risk[254]. Only four of them suggested there might be a positive link, with the review's conclusion being that they didn't think there was enough evidence overall to say if there was a link or not.

Since then, there have been a couple more smaller studies published[255,256], one showing an association between SSB con-sumption and prostate cancer risk specifically, and the other showing an association with breast cancer incidence (in postmeno-pausal women). When we look at research like this it's important to see if there are other factors that might be responsible for the link. People who drink more SSBs have been found to be more likely to smoke, have reduced levels of physical activity and drink more alcohol. Seeing as we *know* that these can all have negative effects on cancer risk, it's certainly not unreasonable to suggest that these might be the culprits as opposed to the SSBs.

One recent larger study showed a link between SSB consumption and overall cancer risk even after attempting to account for these lifestyle factors in their statistical analysis[257]. It had a large sample size, with just over 100,000 participants, but 79 per cent were women and all from France; are those factors? If we look at a study from Australia, we find the exact opposite, with research looking at 35,000 middle-aged Australians over a 19-year period finding no link at all[258]. My point here is that there is a *lot* of conflicting research on the topic, which suggests there are factors at play we're not looking at.

At most we have an association between certain kinds of cancer and sugar-sweetened beverages (not sugar directly), yet that is hugely complicated by the presence of different lifestyle factors that are impossible to fully remove from the statistics. It's one of many reasons why the American Institute for Cancer Research, Cancer Research UK, Mayo Clinic and many other respected global medical institutions agree – sugar doesn't cause cancer.

There are less problematic and more logical reasons to moderate the consumption of added sugar than a fear of cancer (see page 96). 'Moderation through fear' is just a fancy term for restriction. It has a habit of ruining your relationship with food and your health.

'SUGAR FEEDS CANCER'

Although technically true, the fact is that sugar feeds all cells. This lack of scientific understanding has resulted in this statement being used to fear-monger sugar intake. There is no evidence that reducing sugar has any benefit on cancer outcomes.

Pretty much every single cell in our body, including cancer when it happens to occur, uses glucose as a source of energy. With cancer cells growing much faster than everything else they plough through lots of glucose, leaving the rest of our body struggling for energy. This is one of the reasons why people with cancer commonly experience weight loss. As such, you could say the claim that 'sugar feeds cancer' is technically true, but it's *not* true that cutting out sugar/carbs from the diet slows down growth or improves survival rates. We've been researching different ways of curing cancer for decades; do you really think if it worked, we'd be hiding it?

If the restriction of sugar could limit the ability of the cancer cells to grow, most people would take that over chemotherapy any day of the week, but our body is more complicated than that. First, cancer is particularly good at getting hold of even small amounts of available glucose, meaning our normal cells that also need it are actually likely to end up losing out. Second, our body has the ability to make glucose from both fat and protein. This has been shown by the fact that cancer patients following a very low-carbohydrate diet don't show a reduction in blood glucose levels at all[259]. Any attempts at sugar restriction don't actually stop glucose getting to cancer cells like we'd want it to.

If sugar truly *did* 'feed cancer' then it would follow that any drug that increases blood glucose levels would help cancer to grow, right? Enter steroids stage left. These drugs are commonly used as part of cancer therapy to help destroy cancer cells and make chemotherapy more effective, while at the same time *increasing* blood glucose levels.

Research backs all of this up. Several recent systematic reviews[259–261] have not shown *any* benefit to restricting carbohydrates or sugar in patients with cancer. The evidence just isn't there for the claims being made.

A final word of caution: any restrictive dieting while dealing with cancer has the very real potential for unintended weight loss. It can be difficult to eat enough calories anyway while going through cancer treatment, and as such, patients are particularly susceptible to malnutrition. This isn't a risk to be sniffed at. With several studies showing unexpected weight loss in cancer patients when given sugar-restricted diets[260], it's not only pointless but also dangerous.

'ALKALINE DIETS CURE CANCER'

This claim is complete nonsense, yet incredibly prevalent. How many of you have read or heard the following:

> 'No disease, including cancer, can exist in an alkaline environment.'

That quote, attributed to German physiologist, medical doctor and Nobel Prize winner Dr Otto Warburg, is used widely in memes across the internet to justify the claim that alkaline diets are the key to curing cancer. Not only is the claim completely crap but there's absolutely no evidence that he even said it!

Dr Warburg was the first to observe, among other things, that cancer cells produce significant quantities of lactic acid[262]. To appreciate why this happens we need to understand that cells have two options when it comes to producing energy: they can do so with or without oxygen. Producing energy with oxygen, known as aerobic respiration, tends to be the preferred choice as it produces more energy overall. The alternative, known as anaerobic respiration, produces relatively less energy and also results in lactic acid formation.

Cancer cells, for a multitude of different reasons, choose to use anaerobic respiration even when there's lots of oxygen around, hence why Warburg found them to produce lactic acid. The immediate environment around cancer cells therefore becomes acidic, leading some people to claim this means that acidity causes cancer and alkalinity cures it. Let me paint you an analogy . . . it might sound weird at first but stay with me! When it rains, the ground gets wet. If someone tried to tell you that it's actually the ground being wet that causes it to rain, you'd realise they have zero understanding as to how the weather works. This is the same flawed logic as the claim that acidity causes cancer; cancer is what leads to the localised acidity, not the other way around.

As we've already touched on (see page 180), the pH of our body isn't arbitrary. For our cells to function properly their pH

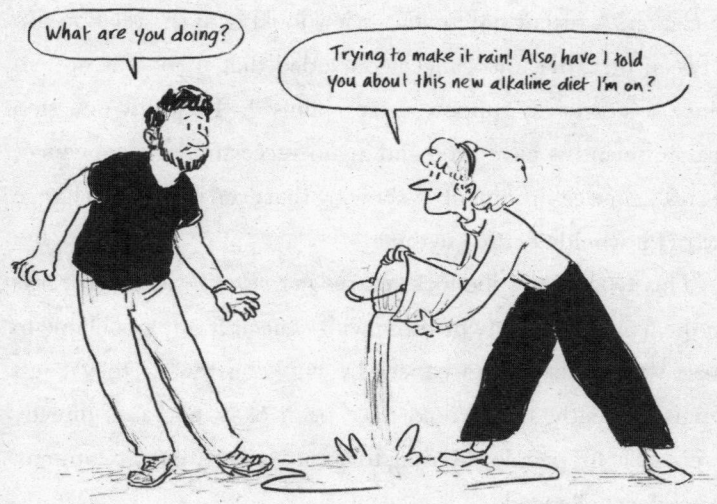

needs to be kept between 7.0 and 7.4, otherwise certain chemical reactions can't take place. Our blood has an even tighter working range, with it being kept between 7.35 and 7.45. Seeing as these are both higher than a neutral pH of 7, it means that our blood and cells are actually both already slightly alkaline. The ridiculous irony of this whole conversation is that the pH inside cancer cells is not only alkaline as well, but actually more alkaline than the pH in our normal ones[263]!

Food can't change the pH of your cells

Now the argument from the charlatans is that certain foods can make your blood 'too acidic', leading to cancer, and an alkaline diet will cure it. This is complete bullshit and the science couldn't be clearer. A recent systematic review looking at the relationship between diet, pH and cancer concluded that there was no evidence *whatsoever* to support these claims[264]. Taking it one step further, scientists have time and again successfully grown cancer in an alkaline environment[265], showing that even if we *could* change the pH it wouldn't cure anything!

This type of nutribollocks makes me *incredibly* angry. It preys on the fear and anxiety of those with cancer. It imparts blame to those who've died from cancer by implying that if they'd just eaten differently, they would have been okay, and it is directly responsible for people choosing to ignore conventional treatment. It *must* be challenged.

Alkaline water is the same nonsense

I'm not sure what came first, alkaline diets or alkaline water, but they're two sides of the same coin. Not only is it frustratingly easy to find bottles of alkaline water in the shops, but you can also buy machines that filter and alkalise your tap water at home. It's not uncommon to find the latter being sold for the absolute *bargain* price of up to £5,000. Let me give you a list of things this privileged water claims to be able to do:

- reverse ageing
- support the immune system
- cause weight loss (because obviously no list would be complete without that one)

- cure cancer
- detox the body
- fix hair loss
- cure osteoporosis
- prevent kidney stones

Literally none of these are true.

Not only that, but a worrying number of the companies selling these machines are predatory pyramid schemes, where people are tricked into 'joining the business' and buying several machines to sell to friends and family. Alkaline water is simply a continuation of the unscientific nonsense behind alkaline diets. It's no different to normal water when it comes to your health.

For the sake of nuance, the only potential benefit from alkaline water *might* be in the improvement of acid reflux symptoms. One study in the lab has shown a particularly alkaline pH of 8.8 may have some benefit[266] (although most bottled alkaline water you can buy is nowhere near that), but there isn't any actual research on people with the condition showing any symptomatic relief. With regular consumption of alkaline water being reported to cause untoward gastrointestinal symptoms and the World Health Organization actually advising against consuming it regularly[267], there are other much safer, cheaper and more reliable ways to manage symptoms of heartburn. Save your money.

'ARTIFICIAL SWEETENERS CAUSE CANCER'

If you spend too much time listening to the wellness gurus of the internet, you'll start to believe that artificial sweeteners are the worst thing since gluten. I promise you that they're not. I've already covered earlier on how they aren't harmful for you (see pages 108–110), but let's look specifically at the cancer claim.

One of the specific concerns revolves around aspartame, most famous for being the sweet taste in Diet Coke. After being broken down by the body it leads to the production of a small amount of formaldehyde, which is known to be able to cause cancer and is used to embalm dead bodies. Wait a second . . . how do we reconcile *that* with the fact we have research saying there's no evidence for aspartame causing cancer[268]?

Well, context is really important. Your body actually produces over 1,000 times more formaldehyde on a typical day than results from a can of Diet Coke. It gets broken down into amino acids (used to make protein), with anything left over being excreted in your urine. A single glass of fruit juice leads to your body making more than five times the amount of formaldehyde than a can of Diet Coke . . . but you don't hear of fruit juice causing cancer now do you? (Well, actually some people might say that, but I refuse to Google it as I'll just end up getting angry.) Unless you're drinking embalming solution or windscreen washer fluid (neither of which I recommend you do) formaldehyde is not something you need to worry about, especially not as a result of aspartame.

How about the other artificial sweeteners? Two different reviews of the available (but limited) research have attempted to answer the question[269,270], with neither finding a positive link. Cancer Research UK is also pretty clear with its stance that artificial sweeteners don't increase the risk of cancer[271].

Cancer risk is the absolute last thing that should be on your mind when someone offers you a Diet Coke.

'RED AND PROCESSED MEAT GIVES YOU CANCER'

Back in 2015 the World Health Organization's International Agency for Research on Cancer (IARC) classified processed meat as a Group 1 carcinogen and red meat as a Group 2A carcinogen. Headlines claiming that bacon was 'as bad for you as smoking' ran in many of the less trustworthy but still widely read newspapers, leading to a fair bit of panic. The lack of understanding as to what the IARC classification actually meant led to many different responses, but my favourite still has to be the following, from the comment section of an online newspaper:

'If scientists think they can take away my bacon they can think again!'

The IARC is an international agency that, in their own words, exists to 'provide the evidence-base for cancer prevention'. As part of their work, they put things into groups depending on how much research there is about their ability to cause cancer.

Group 1:	The agent is carcinogenic to humans.
Group 2A:	The agent is probably carcinogenic to humans.
Group 2B:	The agent is possibly carcinogenic to humans.
Group 3:	The agent is not classifiable as to its carcinogenicity to humans.
Group 4:	The agent is probably not carcinogenic to humans.

The word 'agent' here covers many different things including drugs, radiation, viruses, food, and occupation and lifestyle factors. The groups they are put in only express their impression of certainty, not actual risk. For example, both active and passive smoking (second-hand) are in group 1, yet it's pretty clear that these two are not the same. Both still have the ability to cause cancer, but the risk from active smoking is much greater.

Risk is a funny concept. We tend to over- or underestimate risk as a result of our lived experiences. Sometimes it's not that our estimation is necessarily off, but that the value we choose to put on it differs from someone else's. To use one example: in many European countries the number of healthcare professionals choosing to smoke is higher than that of the general population[272]. We can be relatively safe in assuming that healthcare professionals understand the risks associated with smoking, so what is it that leads them to do so? If you want my honest opinion, I believe that it's a result of working in a profession that exposes us to so much illness every day. This has the potential to generate a numbness to our own personal health risk. Whatever the actual reason (and I'm sure there's more than just one) I think it's both fascinating and a fair bit concerning.

So, how should we be thinking about cancer? Solar radiation is a group 1 carcinogen, but does that mean we should never go outside? Definitely not, as staying indoors for our whole life is far more harmful to our health in the long run and we can reduce our risk by applying sunscreen when necessary. That doesn't mean we should be blasé about these kinds of risks either, but there is definitely a sensible middle ground to aim for.

Let's start with processed meat. This includes things such as bacon, sausages, salami and ham. The IARC agency classified processed meat as a Group 1 carcinogen in 2015 after a range of different types of research showed that it increased the risk of colorectal cancer. It's believed this is due to the presence of compounds called nitrites that are added during processing.

Eating 50g of processed meat each day (about one and a half slices of bacon) leads to an estimated 18 per cent higher *relative* risk of colorectal cancer[273]. That automatically sounds like a scary number, but remember how I talked about how difficult it can be to understand risk? Your *absolute* lifetime risk of being diagnosed with colorectal cancer starts at roughly 5 per cent. An 18 per cent *relative* increase puts that up to 6 per cent. The difference between relative and absolute risk can be confusing and the use of the former is often why the headlines sound scary.

Although I think fear is the wrong emotion, this increase of absolute risk is significant enough that we should still take it seriously; in a population the size of the UK it would equate to over half a million more people with colorectal cancer. I'll leave you with the general advice that although you don't have to remove it from your diet completely, cutting down on processed meat is undeniably a sensible idea.

The conversation around other red meat (steaks etc) is less straightforward.

The IARC have classified it as a Group 2A carcinogen, meaning that they believe it to be 'probably carcinogenic to humans'. Research has consistently found an association between red meat consumption and a higher risk of cancer. On top of that there have been potential mechanisms identified as to how the two might be linked.

At the moment there isn't definitively a causal relationship. What I mean by that is although there has been an association found between red meat and colorectal cancer, whether it is actually *causing* it is less straightforward. Research has shown that, in general, those who consume the most red meat have a lower fibre intake and are more likely to smoke[274]. With fibre able to mediate the risk of colorectal cancer and smoking able to increase it outright, it's difficult to fully remove these factors from the analysis.

Having said that, there is certainly enough evidence to conclude that reducing red meat consumption is a good idea for health, even if you eat lots of fruit and vegetables. Exactly how much red meat is recommended per week varies depending on which country you get the advice from, but you definitely shouldn't be following a carnivore diet.

'DAIRY CAUSES CANCER'

The story of how dairy initially got entangled with cancer is a good example of how our desire to find solutions to our own health can lead us down a route of wanting food to be medicine. It also shows how even the smartest among us can be misled by confirmation bias (see page 188).

Professor Jane Plant, professor of geochemistry at Imperial College London and the chief scientist at the British Geological Survey, was first diagnosed with breast cancer in 1987. During the course of her lifetime she had to deal with its recurrence an unfathomable eight times. In 1993, after the fifth time of it coming back, she read about the low rates of breast cancer in rural Chinese women and hypothesised this to be due to the lack of dairy in their diet. This was a really odd conclusion, especially as there are many other plausible reasons as to why Chinese women have lower rates of breast cancer. They not only consume a lot less alcohol than we do in the UK (something we know to reduce breast cancer risk[275]), but are more likely to have children at a younger age, a protective factor for breast cancer that we've known for the last 50 years[276]. Lastly, rural China has much less access to breast cancer screening. If you simply don't diagnose the cancer that exists the rates are always going to appear lower.

Despite all of this, Jane chose to cut all dairy from her diet and within 12 months her cancer was once again in remission. Even though she was on chemotherapy that whole time, confirmation bias led her down a route of searching for reasons why dairy *must* have been the problem. Her conclusions were as follows:

- The consumption of dairy acidifies the body and therefore increases the risk of cancer. We know this is complete nonsense. As we've already covered (see page 215), food simply cannot change the pH of your body in this way.
- Milk contains a hormone called IGF-1 (insulin-like growth factor 1) that causes breast cancer.

The second theory is a bit more logical than the first, but it still doesn't hold up to scrutiny. Let's start with the facts: milk *does* contain IGF-1, something that has been studied for its role in cancer cell growth[277]. From the outset this seems pretty damning, but like most things in medicine there's a lot more to it. We produce IGF-1 from pretty much every tissue in our body due to the fact that it plays an important role in encouraging our cells to grow and divide; as such there is a quite a bit circulating in our blood at all times. Cancer is incredibly good at surviving and has recognised that it can use this to its benefit. However, just like we covered with sugar, the fact that cancer uses a substance for its benefit is not the same as that substance causing it in the first place.

So, does IGF-1 in dairy cause breast cancer? Well not only does a glass of milk contain less than 0.015 per cent of the IGF-1 your body already produces on a daily basis[278], but it turns out that your gut breaks down the IGF-1 consumed anyway, meaning that we never even end up absorbing it[279].

Despite neither of Jane's theories holding water, her position as someone of scientific authority enabled her to publish a duo of books in the early 2000s claiming you could prevent and treat breast cancer with a non-dairy diet. The fact that she never rejected conventional therapy and was on chemotherapy during her dietary change seemed to be lost on those who bought into her narrative.

In the years since her books were published, a newer argument for the connection between dairy and cancer has arisen, so let's take a quick look and debunk that too.

Breast cancer risk is influenced by one of the main sex hormones, oestrogen. To simplify a relatively complicated topic, both higher exposure to oestrogen over the course of a lifetime, and higher levels after the menopause, can increase breast cancer risk[280]. Add to this the fact that all milk contains small amounts of oestrogen and we have a reason to fear-monger dairy again! Fortunately, this isn't actually a cause for concern at all. A glass of whole milk contains 28,000 times *less* oestrogen than the female body normally produces in a day. This is an absolutely pitiful amount and way too little to have any physiological effect on breast tissue[281].

The evidence simply doesn't exist to back up the claim that dairy causes cancer[282], no matter which argument someone is using. In fact, if anything, milk consumption has actually been shown to be associated with a *lower* risk of colorectal cancer[283]. Dairy can be a fantastic source of calcium and is often people's main source of iodine, which is incredibly important for thyroid function. We need to stop demonising it.

'FASTING PREVENTS / CURES CANCER'

We already started covering the topic of autophagy and intermittent fasting back on page 167, but now let's look at the discussion in relation to cancer.

To recap briefly, autophagy is a process that primarily functions to renew and maintain cells so they don't have to be replaced, but can also promote cell death[284] when required. It also helps to recycle parts of the cell for use elsewhere in the body under stress conditions like nutrient starvation[196].

The role of autophagy in cancer has been investigated extensively. With damage to our cells having the potential to increase the risk of cancer, autophagy is one of the many mechanisms in place to protect against this. However, the consensus at present is that it appears to play a dual and opposite role in both cancer suppression and cancer promotion depending on the type and stage of tumour[285]. If you were able to reliably boost the process of autophagy in your body (which you can't), it wouldn't be a particularly advisable choice – you may actually end up *increasing* your risk of certain cancers!

Enter fasting. The theory is that stimulating autophagy by not eating for a prolonged period of time will both prevent cancer formation and treat already established cancer. Let's be very clear; there's no good evidence that encouraging autophagy in the context of human starvation does anything more than just recycle nutrients. It isn't going to prevent or cure cancer. Not only would it have to increase the other functions of autophagy, but it could actually have the potential to increase the risk of cancer, so this theory is rubbish. Autophagy is a crucial process in the body, but more of a good thing is not always better!

Those telling you to starve yourself for health will often throw a few studies done in mice and parasitic worms at you to try to prove that they're right. The reason why they can't quote human studies is because 'it remains practically impossible to monitor autophagy properly in humans[197]'. If science can't monitor it yet it seems even more ridiculous that so many claims about it are being made with such confidence!

A common question I like to ask those who encourage fasting is why they don't also promote the other things that we know that increase autophagy. Exercise[286] and good sleep[287] both increase it, but I'd imagine it's a lot harder to make money from them than it is from a fasting regime. If you want to see their mind explode, it's also fun to tell that them that sleep *deprivation* has also been shown to increase autophagy[288]. So, all we've got to do is starve ourselves while exercising and make sure we get good sleep and bad sleep? If you're going to be unscientific at least be consistent about it . . .

To end on a more nuanced note, there has been some interesting research into whether fasting may improve the side effects of chemotherapy and radiotherapy, with a few different studies showing promising results[289]. Important to note here that not only were these small studies, some with as few as six patients, but they were trialling long fasting periods of five days back-to-back. Not trivial.

It's really important to acknowledge that deliberate fasting during cancer has a big potential for unintended weight loss. It can be difficult to eat enough calories anyway while going through cancer treatment due to things like nausea and loss of appetite, as such patients are particularly susceptible to malnutrition. The studies mentioned above were unable to get ethical approval for full fasting as a result of this, so they instead mimicked it as much as possible by having patients consume very low-calorie diets. They were also under incredibly tight supervision from oncology doctors and dietitians. Fasting is likely to be really harmful for a large proportion of the population with cancer, so please don't think of this as a valid option without having a frank discussion with your doctor.

'JUICING CURES CANCER'

One of the most heartbreaking things to see on social media are posts documenting the difficulties that a young child has to deal with after a diagnosis of cancer such as leukaemia. Equally heartbreaking is the fact that it's becoming increasingly common to see parents giving their children juicing regimes in a distressing attempt to cure.

Whenever I come across one of these accounts my heart sits in my throat as I scan through some of the recent posts. More often than not there'll be a picture of the child being given celery juice to sip through a straw. Have you noticed how the price of celery has skyrocketed in the last couple of years? This is a direct result of Anthony William, a.k.a the Medical Medium.

He claims to have been 'born with the unique ability to

converse with the Spirit of Compassion, who provides him with extraordinarily accurate health information that's far ahead of its time. Since age four, Anthony has been using his gift to read people's conditions and tell them how to recover their health.' I promise I'm not making this crap up; that's copied directly from his website[290]. He talks to a 'spirit' that gives him health knowledge that conveniently can't be debunked because it's so ahead of it's time that doctors just haven't discovered yet. Eugh.

Most people claiming blatant nutribollocks like this don't gain much traction, but for some reason he's gained a cult-like following from a slew of celebrities including Sylvester Stallone, Pharrell Williams, Gwyneth Paltrow and Miranda Kerr, as well as over seven million followers on social media and an appearance on *Keeping Up*

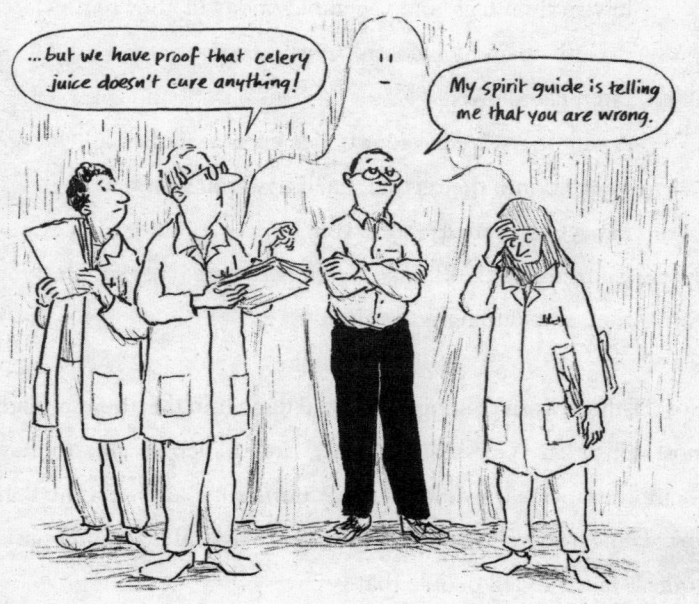

With The Kardashians. His book on celery juice[291] claims that it is 'one of the most profound, preventative anti-cancer herbs' and even gives recommended quantities for someone 'trying to prevent or cope with cancer'. It's utterly terrifying that this was even allowed to be published. In case you were wondering, he's making all of this up.

Although the Medical Medium is responsible for the current boom in popularity, the concept of juicing in order to cure ailments seems to have originated back in the 1920s with German doctor Max Gerson. What started as a supposed cure for migraine headaches morphed into a treatment for cancer and came to be known as Gerson Therapy or the Gerson Diet. The rules are a scary mix of privilege and serious harm:

- Eat 9kg of juiced, organic, high-potassium and low-sodium fruit and vegetables a day (if they're not organic the magic doesn't work, clearly)
- No meat allowed
- Administer three to four coffee enemas (coffee injected into the rectum) each day. You weren't expecting that one, were you?!
- To round it all off, take a concoction of daily supplements (including potassium)

Now, if there wasn't enough potential danger in the above already, most self-titled 'Gerson therapists' advise people not to have chemotherapy as it would 'damage immunity' and ruin the therapy. Dangerous charlatans. Even the Medical Medium hasn't gone as far as to tell people that yet.

Gerson advocates claim, with absolutely zero evidence to back it up, that fruit and vegetables cleanse and/or detox the liver. This is simply not true. The only thing that comes close to doing that is cutting out all alcohol from your diet. You can usually tell someone doesn't know what they're on about when they start using the words 'cleanse' or 'detox', as these words mean absolutely nothing in the context of food. Despite fruit and veg being good for you, consuming that much each day doesn't leave room for much else. It would be pretty easy to become malnourished from the lack of protein – not a state you want to be in while your body is trying to fight cancer.

The coffee enemas are potentially very harmful, especially with how frequently they're advised. Enemas can cause constipation and colitis (inflammation of the bowel) if used regularly. The claim that they detox the colon is also nonsense. The best way to improve the health of your colon is, ironically, to increase fruit and veg consumption . . . but don't remove all the fibre by juicing it all!

The focus on potassium is due to the fact they believe cancer is caused by having too much sodium (salt) in comparison to potassium. Not only is this complete nonsense, but it's where the definite harm starts. If you consume so much potassium that your kidneys can't get rid of it fast enough (which is completely possible through over-supplementation), you end up with a real risk of palpitations, cardiac arrhythmias and sudden cardiac death. Not something to be messing around with.

In case all of that wasn't enough to convince you, research looking at the diet back in 2014 found absolutely no evidence that it had any benefit for cancer[228].

I'm really happy to say that I haven't yet seen any children with cancer being given coffee enemas. However, the fact that there are so many parents being tricked into starting them on juicing regimes and rejecting conventional therapy fills my heart with dread and is one of the many reasons why I keep fighting against this stuff.

'ORGANIC FOOD REDUCES CANCER RISK'

No, it doesn't. Those who choose to buy organic food are more likely to engage in healthy lifestyle behaviours and be from a higher socio-economic class. Both of these independently reduce their risk of cancer.

The topic of organic food is one of privilege. Let me explain what I mean by that. For those of you who enjoy spending your money on organic food and are currently picking up your pitchforks, let me ask you *why* you choose to do that? The most likely reason is that someone told you it was healthier . . . but is it? Despite organic food becoming cheaper in recent years it is still substantially more expensive than buying the conventional option, so let me do you the honour of empowering your wallet with a simple fact:

There is absolutely no evidence that organic food is any safer or healthier than the conventional alternative[292].

Having said that, a recent study[293] found that people who ate the most organic food had a 24 per cent lower risk of developing cancer compared to those who ate the least. Let's explain. The study looked at 69,000 middle-aged French adults (78 per cent women) from the NutriNet-Santé cohort and compared their organic food intake with risk of cancer over a period of five years. The 24 per cent reduction in risk that they found with high organic food intake seems convincing, but there are some pretty good reasons why this doesn't show causation.

People who buy organic food are, on average, more likely to engage in healthy lifestyle behaviours. The study above found this to be the case, with those reporting eating more organic food also exercising more, smoking less and having a diet higher in fibre, vegetables and nutrients. All of these individually have the ability to positively affect cancer risk.

The study attempted to remove these factors in the statistical analysis, but here's the thing about lifestyle – it's complex. The authors of the study even acknowledged in their conclusions that they weren't able to adjust for everything. Now, this is often the case for the vast majority of studies looking at health, so why is this one particularly lacking?

In my opinion it comes down to socio-economics. The ability to afford organic food in the first place requires a certain amount of disposable income; those in the study reporting eating more organic food had both a higher monthly income and higher occupational status. We know that poverty itself is a risk factor for cancer[294,295] and it's next to impossible to be able to control for all the variables that brings with it.

Studies in different countries have found absolutely no association between organic food intake and overall cancer incidence[296]. This means that I'm going to have to agree with both the

American Institute for Cancer Research and Cancer Research UK when they say that organic food hasn't been shown to reduce the risk of cancer. Based on all the evidence so far, including the fact that organic food is mostly pointless from a health perspective anyway, I don't think this is going to change any time soon.

'PESTICIDES GIVE YOU CANCER'

Hold up one second. This isn't true? Are you telling me that pesticides don't cause cancer?!

That's exactly what I'm telling you. There is an awful lot of fear surrounding the discussion of pesticides as they've become synonymous with the words 'unnatural' and 'toxic'. Pretty much everything on earth can be poisonous depending on how much we're exposed to; even water can kill us if we drink too much. Sounds like a silly example? Let me give you a better one.

Glyphosate, the world's most widely used weedkiller, is over 30 times less toxic for you than caffeine, yet you don't fear your morning coffee. The quantities of pesticides that we consume as a result of conventional farming are so far below the toxic threshold it's silly. They categorically have no negative impact on our health.

It's important to note that organic farming *also* uses pesticides (ones that plants produce in an attempt to survive being eaten). These 'natural' ones have to be used in larger quantities seeing as they don't work as well, meaning that on a daily basis we consume 10,000 times more of these than we do the synthetic variety[297].

Good thing they're all perfectly safe as well! None of the plants we consume on a daily basis, whether they be organic or conventional, lead to us developing cancer.

To burst another bubble right at the very end, the argument that organic food is always more sustainable for the environment isn't true either, seeing as organic farming often ends up producing less food and therefore requires more land to get the same yield.

'SOY CAUSES BREAST CANCER'

From a nutritional standpoint soy is pretty amazing. It has been shown to modestly reduce cholesterol levels and potentially improve other markers of cardiovascular health[298]. Remember, food is not medicine, but it does seem to be a good idea to include soy in a balanced diet: it is a great source of fibre, protein, vitamins, minerals and polyunsaturated fat. With all of this going for it where has the cancer fear come from?

What started off as a misunderstanding of the research has now morphed into a right-wing, racial insult. I don't think anyone could have predicted that one.

Soybean is a legume native to East Asia with an enormous variety of uses. The edamame that you find served at sushi restaurants? Immature soybeans. When left to reach maturity they are used to make soy sauce and tofu, as well as forming the base of many different fermented pastes such as miso.

Soy contains what are known as isoflavones, compounds with

a similar chemical structure to the sex hormone oestrogen. With oestrogen exposure known to increase breast cancer risk[280] there was an initial concern that the consumption of soy might do the same. Multiple rodent studies then added fuel to the fire after showing that human breast cancer cells implanted in mice grew faster when they were fed soy[299].

This is probably a good time to remind you again that you're not a mouse.

Now, I know I'm being a bit facetious here, but we have a habit of reading too much into rodent studies. Mice studies can be very helpful at pointing us in the right direction for further research, but to this day we still jump to conclusions and make statements we shouldn't. It's both hilarious and concerning that a Twitter account called @justsaysinmice exists purely to retweet misleading news articles that make bold claims about rodent research . . . with the important clarification that the research was 'in mice'.

It's been shown since that rodents metabolise isoflavones very differently to us humans[300], with a whole host of other research suggesting that these isoflavones may actually be *protective* for breast cancer[301], particularly when consumed from an early age[298].

There's more we could go into but for now let's be clear: the overwhelming scientific consensus currently is that soy consumption doesn't increase cancer risk.

The second thing to address is how consuming soy became a right-wing, racial insult in the form of the term 'soy boy'. Insecure men now use this to insult other men they consider 'unmanly' because of their different views on immigration policy, climate change and feminism. It's utterly ridiculous. They claim that science is on their side and eating soy makes you less stereotypically 'masculine' by reducing testosterone, but this simply isn't true[302].

In addition to the toxic masculinity, the insult has a foundation in racism. Most babies can digest the lactose sugar in cow's milk without an issue, due to the enzyme lactase. The majority of this enzyme used to disappear when we reached adulthood, but evolution has resulted in certain cultures keeping it. Around a third of the global population[303] now have the ability to drink milk as adults without getting an upset stomach, with the vast majority of those being of Northern and Central European descent. This has led to white nationalist groups chugging cow's milk in a deplorable attempt to prove supremacy over those who aren't able to. The term 'soy boy' takes this one step further and harks back to the colonial-era stereotypes of Asian populations being 'effeminate', 'weaker' and 'intellectually inferior' because they ate more plants than their colonisers[304], just this time using a claim of 'science' in an attempt to gloss over the racism.

With the recent influx of different plant-based products designed to taste like meat (including the Impossible™ Burger made from soy and potato protein), those with a fragile sense of masculinity have put these products of the list of things that make you somehow 'less of a man'. When you hear the term 'soy boy' being used please call it for what it is. Nutribollocks being used to justify racism is a new low.

'ANTIPERSPIRANTS CAUSE BREAST CANCER'

Okay, not food-related, but important, so here's some bonus info.

There's been a bit of a trend in the last decade for 'natural' deodorants/antiperspirants that claim to be healthier for you because they don't cause breast cancer, but is this even a real worry? Breast cancer most commonly occurs in the upper outer quadrant of the breast, the area closest to the armpit. The theory claims that by blocking the sweat ducts with aluminium-based antiperspirants you trap the 'toxins' inside the breast near the armpit, which then build up and cause cancer. Let me be very clear – there's no evidence for this being true[305].

Not only is there no evidence for this 'trapped toxins' claim, but the good news is that we have a pretty good idea as to why breast cancer occurs more frequently in the upper outer quadrant. First, that area actually contains less fat and more breast tissue[306], meaning it's more likely for cancer to occur. Second, it's been found that the breast tissue in this area has what's called 'greater genomic instability'[307], meaning that the DNA of the cells in this area is unfortunately simply more likely to gather mutations that can cause cancer.

Only 0.012 per cent of the aluminium from antiperspirants gets absorbed through the skin[308]. To put that into context, a week's worth of aluminium absorption from antiperspirants is 40 times less than we get from our food in the same time period. One of the main functions of our skin is to be a barrier and keep things out – thankfully it's pretty good at it.

So, purchase whichever deodorant or antiperspirant you want, just please don't buy into the whole aluminium-free health nonsense. It's really not worth the extra money.

Does everything we eat cause cancer?

The simple answer to that question is a resounding no, but there's a reason I bring it up.

An absolutely fascinating study investigated 50 randomly selected ingredients from an old American cookbook to see just how many of them were associated with cancer[309]. It found that a whopping 80 per cent had at least one study that related them to cancer in some way, with almost 40 per cent of those studies concluding that the ingredient increased cancer risk. These weren't weird ingredients either; the list included common items such as flour, potato, tomato, beef and peas.

Cancer is *incredibly* complex and there are many things that

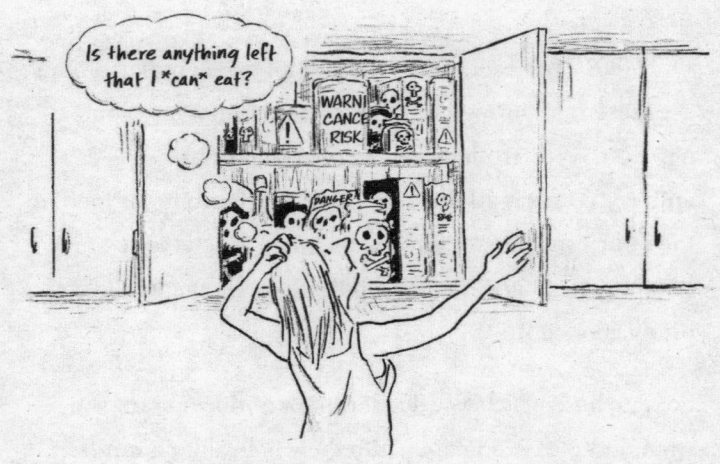

influence its development. This means the results of a study can often be confounded by one of these factors without us realising. Even something as benign as tomatoes can be made to appear cancerous if we cherry-pick one study rather than the breadth of available research.

Keep this at the back of your mind when you come across things online. Even though some individual items can have a bigger impact on our risk of cancer than others, like we see when it comes to processed meat, the biggest deciding factor is our overall eating pattern. Have respect for what food can do without taking it too far. Remember, it's not medicine.

9.

IMPROVING YOUR RELATIONSHIP WITH FOOD

How are you feeling after all that? Are you okay? It can feel incredibly overwhelming to have a lot of your beliefs about health and nutrition challenged in one go, but if it helps, I like to think of it a bit like ripping off a plaster. Why prolong the discomfort?

When you pull off a plaster it's usually with the knowledge that what's underneath is ready to be exposed to the open air. If you're anything like I was when I first started being introduced to how food isn't medicine and weight doesn't define health, it really doesn't *feel* like you're ready does it? Let me speak to those of you who resonate with that for a second.

Spending months or years chasing weight loss, while being exposed to an endless stream of nutribollocks, leads to your relationship with food taking a solid hit. Even when we *aren't* trying to lose weight, our food choices still tend to be based around a fear of fatness disguised under a label of 'health'. When cracks start to form in what we have convinced ourselves is 'right', it can feel like

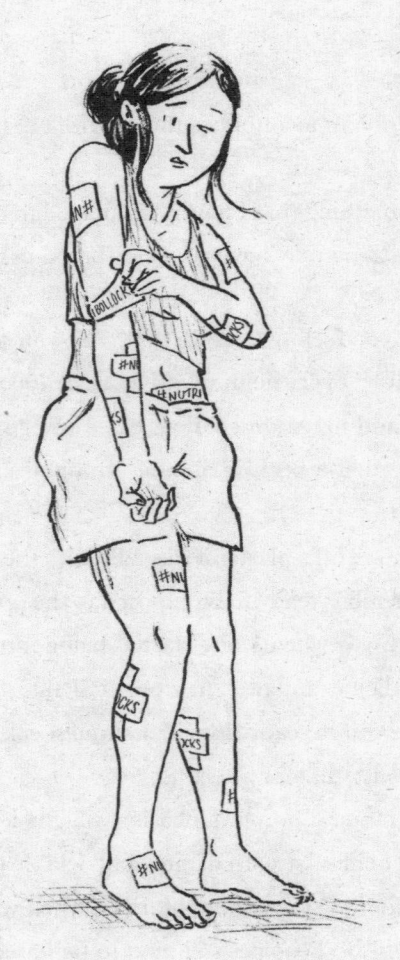

your world is crumbling a little. I've been there. It's worth the discomfort though, I promise.

No matter your background or previous experiences, I'm adamant that one of the first steps to repairing your relationship with food is challenging the misinformation. It's similar to how admitting you're an alcoholic is the essential first step to getting sober.

Is there something that I haven't managed to cover in the previous chapters? You may have a specific belief in mind that hasn't been addressed. I'd like to reassure you with an example that I think should address any remaining worries, and also arm you with an approach to deal with any new nonsense that comes along.

How many of you have been told that we shouldn't be eating carbs after 6pm? I know that I definitely was. The full claim is that eating carbs after 6pm makes you fat . . . and we've covered *in depth* why trying to blame a particular macronutrient for weight gain is near-sighted. Do you really need to know the ins and outs of whether our gut is more efficient at digesting food at different times of the day?

We need to get comfortable at not needing every last detail to challenge something that's otherwise going to negatively impact our relationship with food.

I guarantee that diet culture will always find new ways of trying to draw you in and sell you something. Refusing to eat carbs after 6pm is simply another nonsense rule that is going to be placed on your eating habits. Building a good relationship with food means *fewer* unnecessary rules, not more. A good relationship with food allows you to relax around mealtimes; it allows you to respect the impact that food can have on your health without allowing fear to govern your choices. This all might sound a bit like a lofty ideal, but it's 100 per cent attainable. Don't let anyone lie to you and tell you it's not.

You might now be thinking: 'Great! I had a gut feeling that stuff was a load of nutribollocks all along, but I've believed it for years . . . where do I go from here?' Well, let me introduce you to a few concepts that I believe will help.

Unconditional permission to eat all foods

Are there certain foods that you don't allow yourself to keep in the house due to the fear you'll binge on them? Pringles used to hold that power over me up until very recently. Remember the slogan, 'once you pop, you can't stop'? We tend to forget just how much power words can have. Combine that with my childhood experiences (see page 16) and I would regularly find myself eating them past fullness.

As physical discomfort set in, guilt and shame would follow. That shame would then lead to me setting a rule that I wasn't allowed to buy them anymore as I simply didn't have the will-power to control myself. A couple of weeks later I'd 'accidentally' break my own rule only to end up eating them past fullness again. Does any of that cycle sound familiar?

Today, I'm happy to report that Pringles live in my cupboard as something I'm able to snack on without any overwhelming fear of bingeing. The reason for this change might initially sound counterintuitive, but hear me out: instead of creating more rules as to how much I was allowed to have, I gave myself uncondi-tional permission to eat as many as I wanted.

The concept of 'unconditional permission' when it comes to food freaks people out. It's a predictable response seeing as we live in a society that constantly reinforces a message of restriction and weight loss. The cycle of binge/restriction can't be fixed by just forcing yourself to have more willpower and control. Doing so can even lead to more problems; it's not a coincidence that control is central to many people's experience of eating disorders.

When I first started to try this approach, I still ended up eating the full tube of Pringles, for quite a while. The difference was that the permission I had now given myself meant that the feelings of guilt and shame started to lessen. Over time, I stopped wanting to finish the whole tube as it didn't make me feel good. I actually started being able to *listen* to how my body was feeling and stop short of reaching the point of physical discomfort.

It's pretty clear that eating too many Pringles isn't good for my health; none of this process is arguing against that. The end goal, with building a healthy relationship with food, is to eat *more* nutritious food and be able to moderate things like Pringles. Without unconditional permission to eat however, that attempted moderation always comes from a place of fear.

- Moderation through fear is restriction.
- Restriction worsens health.

Moderation through freedom is a healthy aim. Remember here that I'm talking about moderating less nutritious food, *not* moderating calories to prevent weight gain. That's not health either.

Honouring your hunger

Hunger is the most natural of instincts so why do we insist on finding new ways to ignore it?

When we try to ignore or blunt our hunger, it becomes much harder to make intuitive choices around food. It also becomes difficult to choose nutritious meals when you're ravenous. If our goal is to improve our relationship with food and our health, we need to start honouring our hunger rather than treating it like something unwanted. When you're thirsty, you drink something. When you're hungry, try eating something!

How many times have you heard that 'the parts of the brain that deal with hunger and thirst are very close to each other, so it can be easy to confuse them'? The dieting blogs that push this message never give any real references for where the claim comes from, because it's simply nonsense.

The sensations of hunger and thirst are processed by different mechanisms[310]. It's a good thing too, as we really wouldn't have got very far as a species otherwise. Drinking when hungry just temporarily fills up your stomach and blunts your hunger signals, making it harder to listen to your body in the long run.

We need to stop assuming that our hunger isn't real.

Respecting your fullness

I remember once seeing a child give an ice cream back to their parents halfway through eating it as they didn't want it anymore. That's stuck with me ever since. When was the last time I did that! As adults, it seems almost rude not to finish something, yet often it can mean becoming uncomfortably full as a result. It doesn't help that a lot of us also struggle to recognise the fact that we're no longer hungry, until that moment has been and gone.

There are things that can make respecting your fullness easier:

- Try to remove distractions while eating, such as the TV, that can make it harder to listen to how you are feeling. Sitting at the table instead of on the sofa can really help.
- Try making a purposeful effort to slow down and even take short breaks during the meal to check in on how you're feeling.
- Don't be afraid to leave food; you can always eat it later. On the other hand, if you deliberately want to eat past the point of comfortable fullness, I'm not here to condemn you for that either. Sometimes that extra piece of lasagne is simply not going to wait until tomorrow. Remember that the word 'respect' doesn't mean 'obey'; this stuff isn't black and white.

When you start to attempt these things, they may not feel easy at all. Written down on the page it might appear so, but in practice it never is. Your relationship with food isn't something that changes overnight; it takes time and effort. It may even seem to get worse before it gets better . . . but it *will* get better and it is well worth the process, I promise.

What about weight loss?

The difficult truth for many of you is that you're going to have to set aside the desire to lose weight in order to actively repair your relationship with food. Let me explain why. If you only give yourself permission to eat when you've decided it fits with your weight-loss goals, the permission isn't unconditional. It only becomes possible to truly honour your hunger if you haven't gone over your self-imposed calories for the day. The principle of respecting your fullness gets turned into an excuse not to eat even when you're not actually full. I say this from personal experience not condemnation; my world still revolved around weight loss when I was first introduced to these principles.

I'm not here to condemn people who want to lose weight; I'm just here to remind you that it's neither a risk-free endeavour nor something that defines your health (see chapter 2). Focus on repairing your relationship with food first and foremost. What you do afterwards is your choice, but trying to do both at the same time doesn't work.

Intuitive eating

The principles I've just described are from Intuitive Eating[311]; a flexible framework of principles that can be thought of as a clinical intervention for repairing someone's relationship with food.

Its purpose is to help people get back in tune with the natural signals of hunger, fullness and satisfaction, while still recognising the importance of nutrition for health.

Note, it is *not* a weight-loss diet. Some people find that their body weight shifts closer to their natural setpoint (see page 55) as they get better at listening to their body, but this is neither a guarantee, nor the point. That shift could also mean weight gain.

Since its creation in 1995 there has been a substantial amount of encouraging research around its use, showing Intuitive Eating to improve both psychological and physical health[312] and reduce disordered eating behaviours such as binge eating[313]. It's important to acknowledge that having the ability to fully implement every principle does benefit from a certain amount of socioeconomic privilege. Despite that, I believe the framework is flexible enough for the vast majority of people to benefit.

If this idea of giving yourself unconditional permission to eat and becoming more in tune with hunger and fullness has resonated with you, I strongly recommend that you take some time to explore the full framework in more depth (see Further Resources, page 255).

Moving forward

After all of that we come back to the main purpose of this book: to help you to sift through and identify nutribollocks. To sum up:

1. Food isn't medicine

I had to start with this one, didn't I? If you read something online that tells you that oranges cure breast cancer (or anything else I haven't specifically talked about in this book) you can rest assured that it's likely to be utter nonsense. The misconception that food is medicine makes it much easier to believe that a lot of the nutribollocks could be true, so it's incredibly important to challenge this first and foremost.

2. *Everything in moderation*

If the advice you're being given doesn't recognise this fact, throw it out. Some foods are better for your health than others, but that doesn't mean that we should demonise any of them. The best example of this is when you come across someone who tells you to remove an entire food group from your diet. It's completely unnecessary and has great potential to ruin your relationship with food. Focus on repairing that relationship so that you are able to moderate from a place of freedom rather than fear.

3. *There is no 'best' diet for weight loss*

The vast majority of nutritional advice tends to come with a promise of weight loss in some form or another (I'm looking at you, keto). Every month someone new claims to have found the solution (often a medical doctor capitalising on the incorrect assumption that weight and health are synonymous in order to make money from a book). There is no magical diet that will supersede the multifactorial nature of body size. If someone claims to have found one, they are ignorant or simply lying to you.

So, what does a 'healthy' diet look like then? I consider myself to be a nutritional agnostic, meaning that I believe different people have different nutritional needs. A healthy diet can look different depending on who you are talking to and what else is going on in their life, at that moment in time. Acknowledging that, we can look at the healthiest eating pattern, in general, when all else is equal. Remember always that people's access to food is hugely impacted by inequity and socio-economics (see page 36) and we should never shame ourselves or others for not being able to follow this to the letter. The following short guidelines tend to hold true:

- Eat more vegetables and fruits
- Eat more sources of fibre (grains, seeds, nuts, beans and legumes)
- Include oily fish, lean white meat, eggs and plant sources of protein (such as tofu)
- Include both olive and rapeseed oil (extra virgin if you can afford it)
- Include dairy (yoghurt, milk and cheese)
- Eat less sugar, saturated fat, and red and processed meat

When it comes to food, your health is impacted by your dietary pattern over a period of time. Don't you dare beat yourself up if there are days when all you eat are crisps, dip and mince pies. Those are sometimes the best days. Instead, focus on inclusion rather than exclusion. Including more nutritious food rather than trying to exclude the less nutritious items is going to both improve your health *and* benefit your relationship with food. Win-win. There's no benefit in choosing the objectively healthier option for dinner if you're doing it from a place of guilt and shame.

Not only do morals have no place when it comes to food, but trying to change behaviour that way simply doesn't work.

Further Resources

Books

HAES

Health at Every Size: The Surprising Truth About Your Weight by Linda Bacon, PhD
Radical Belonging: How to Survive and Thrive in an Unjust World (While Transforming it for the Better) by Lindo Bacon, PhD

Nutrition

Is Butter a Carb?: Unpicking Fact from Fiction in the World of Nutrition by Rosie Saunt and Helen West
The Angry Chef: Bad Science and the Truth About Healthy Eating by Anthony Warner
The No Need to Diet Book: Become a Diet Rebel and Make Friends with Food by Pixie Turner

Intuitive Eating

Intuitive Eating: A Revolutionary Anti-Diet Approach by Evelyn Tribole and Elyse Resch
Just Eat It: How Intuitive Eating Can Help You Get Your Shit Together Around Food by Laura Thomas, PhD
Train Happy: An Intuitive Exercise Plan for Every Body by Tally Rye

Science/Socio-economics

Bad Science by Ben Goldacre
The Health Gap: The Challenge of an Unequal World by Michael Marmot

Websites

HAES/Intuitive Eating

https://asdah.org
https://lindobacon.com/_resources/
https://www.intuitiveeating.org

Nutrition

https://www.alineanutrition.com/

Eating Disorders

https://www.beateatingdisorders.org.uk
https://www.nationaleatingdisorders.org

Podcasts

Cut Through Nutrition – Dr Joshua Wolrich & Alan Flanagan
Don't Salt My Game – Laura Thomas, PhD
Food Psych Podcast – Christy Harrison
In Bad Taste – Pixie Turner and Nikki Stamp
Nutrition Matters Podcast – Paige Smathers
Unpacking Weight Science – Fiona Willer
Willing to be Wrong – Dr Joshua Wolrich

References

1. Marton RM, Wang X, Barabási A-L & Ioannidis JPA. 'Science, advocacy, and quackery in nutritional books: an analysis of conflicting advice and purported claims of nutritional best-sellers.' Palgrave Communications 6 (2020) 1–6

2. Cardenas D. 'Let not thy food be confused with thy medicine: The Hippocratic misquotation.' e-SPEN Journal 8 (2013) e260–e262

3. Blair Bell W. 'Menstruation and its relationship to the calcium metabolism.' Proceedings of the Royal Society of Medicine 1 (1908) 291–314

4. Bacon L. *Health at every size: The surprising truth about your weight* (BenBella Books, Inc., 2010)

5. The Epidemiology Monitor. 'Highlights From An Australian Interview With Sir Michael Marmot And His Recent Canadian Presentation To Health Economists' (2011). Retrieved from http://epimonitor.net/Michael_Marmot_Interview.htm (accessed Nov 2020)

6. Organisation for Economic Co-operation and Development. 'A Broken Social Elevator? How to Promote Social Mobility.' OECD Publishing (2018) 352

7. Food Foundation. 'The Broken Plate Report' (2019). Retrieved from https://foodfoundation.org.uk/publication/the-broken-plate-report/ (accessed Sept 2020)

8. Corfe S. 'What are the barriers to eating healthily in the UK?' (2018). Retrievedfromhttps://www.smf.co.uk/publications/barriers-eating-healthily-uk (accessed Sept 2020)

9. Turn2us. 'Living Without: The Scale & Impact of Appliance Poverty' (2020). Retrieved from https://www.turn2us.org.uk/About-Us/Our-Campaigns/Living-Without-Campaign/About-the-campaign (accessed Oct 2020)

10. Pampel FC, Denney JT & Krueger PM. 'Obesity, SES, and economic development: a test of the reversal hypothesis.' Social Science & Medicine 74 (2012) 1073–1081

11. Keys A, Fidanza F, Karvonen MJ, Kimura N & Taylor HL. 'Indices of relative weight and obesity.' Journal of Chronic Diseases 25 (1972) 329–343

12. Burton BT, Foster WR, Hirsch J & Van Itallie TB. 'Health implications of obesity: an NIH Consensus Development Conference.' International Journal of Obesity 9 (1985) 155–170

13. Ernsberger P & Koletsky RJ. 'Weight cycling.' JAMA 273 (1995) 998–999

14. Troiano RP, Frongillo EA, Sobal J & Levitsky DA. 'The relationship between body weight and mortality: a quantitative analysis of combined information from existing studies.' International Journal of Obesity and Related Metabolic Disorders 20 (1996) 63–75

15. Bhaskaran K, Dos-Santos-Silva I, Leon DA, Douglas IJ & Smeeth L. 'Association of BMI with overall and cause-specific mortality: a population-based cohort study of 3·6 million adults in the UK.' The Lancet Diabetes & Endocrinology 6 (2018) 944–953

16. Flegal KM, Kit BK, Orpana H & Graubard BI. 'Association of all-cause mortality with overweight and obesity using standard body mass index categories: a systematic review and meta-analysis.' JAMA 309 (2013) 71–82

17. Sutin AR, Stephan Y & Terracciano A. 'Weight Discrimination and Risk of Mortality.' Psychological Science 26 (2015) 1803–1811

18. Gujral UP et al. 'Cardiometabolic abnormalities among normal-weight persons from five racial/ethnic groups in the United States: a cross-sectional analysis of two cohort studies.' Annals of Internal Medicine 166 (2017) 628–636

19. Tomiyama AJ, Hunger JM, Nguyen-Cuu J & Wells C. 'Misclassification of cardiometabolic health when using body mass index categories in NHANES 2005–2012.' International Journal of Obesity 40 (2016) 883–886

20. Coelho M, Oliveira T & Fernandes R. 'Biochemistry of adipose tissue: an endocrine organ.' Archives of Medical Science 9 (2013) 191

21. Hardy OT, Czech MP & Corvera S. 'What causes the insulin resistance underlying obesity.' Current Opinion in Endocrinology Diabetes and Obesity 19 (2012) 81–87

22. Stefan N, Schick F & Häring H-U. 'Causes, characteristics, and consequences of metabolically unhealthy normal weight in humans.' Cell Metabolism 26 (2017) 292–300

23. Vissers D et al. 'The effect of exercise on visceral adipose tissue in overweight adults: a systematic review and meta-analysis.' PLoS One 8 (2013) e56415

24. Sweatt SK, Gower BA, Chieh AY, Liu Y & Li L. 'Sleep quality is differentially related to adiposity in adults.' Psychoneuroendocrinology 98 (2018) 46–51

25. Davis JN, Alexander KE, Ventura EE, Toledo-Corral CM & Goran MI. 'Inverse relation between dietary fiber intake and visceral adiposity in overweight Latino youth.' The American Journal of Clinical Nutrition 90 (2009) 1160–1166

26. Drapeau V, Therrien F, Richard D & Tremblay A. 'Is visceral obesity a physiological adaptation to stress.' Panminerva Medica 45 (2003) 189–196

27. Haleem S, Lutchman L, Mayahi R, Grice JE & Parker MJ. 'Mortality following hip fracture: trends and geographical variations over the last 40 years.' Injury 39 (2008) 1157–1163

28. Chang CS et al. 'Inverse relationship between central obesity and osteoporosis in osteoporotic drug naive elderly females: The Tianliao Old People (TOP) Study.' Journal of Clinical Densitometry 16 (2013) 204–211

29. Meczekalski B, Katulski K, Czyzyk A, Podfigurna-Stopa A & Maciejewska-Jeske M. 'Functional hypothalamic amenorrhea and its influence on women's health.' J Endocrinol Invest 37 (2014) 1049–1056

30. Janice P, Shaffer R, Sinno Z, Tyler M & Ghosh J. 'The obesity paradox in ICU patients.' Annu Int Conf IEEE Eng Med Biol Soc 2017 (2017) 3360–3364

31. Intensive Care National Audit & Research Centre. 'ICNARC report on COVID-19 in critical care 29 May 2020' (2020). Retrieved from https://www.icnarc.org/Our-Audit/Audits/Cmp/Reports (accessed June 2020)

32. Matheson EM, King DE & Everett CJ. 'Healthy lifestyle habits and mortality in overweight and obese individuals.' Journal of the American Board of Family Medicine 25 (2012) 9–15

33. Barry VW et al. 'Fitness vs. fatness on all-cause mortality: a meta-analysis.' Progress in Cardiovasc Diseases 56 (2014) 382–390

34. Anderson JW, Konz EC, Frederich RC & Wood CL. 'Long-term weight-loss maintenance: a meta-analysis of US studies.' The American Journal of Clinical Nutrition 74 (2001) 579–584

35. Wing RR & Phelan S. 'Long-term weight loss maintenance.' The American Journal of Clinical Nutrition 82 (2005) 222S–225S

36. Leibel RL, Rosenbaum M & Hirsch J. 'Changes in energy expenditure resulting from altered body weight.' New England Journal of Medicine 332 (1995) 621–628

37. Kubasova N, Burdakov D & Domingos AI. 'Sweet and Low on Leptin: Hormonal Regulation of Sweet Taste Buds.' Diabetes 64 (2015) 3651–3652

38. Wadden TA et al. 'Short- and long-term changes in serum leptin dieting obese women: effects of caloric restriction and weight loss.' The Journal of Clinical Endocrinology and Metabolism 83 (1998) 214–218

39. Gruzdeva O, Borodkina D, Uchasova E, Dyleva Y & Barbarash O. 'Leptin resistance: underlying mechanisms and diagnosis.' Diabetes Metabolic Syndrome and Obesity 12 (2019) 191–198

40. Lowe MR, Doshi SD, Katterman SN & Feig EH. 'Dieting and restrained eating as prospective predictors of weight gain.' Frontiers in Psychology 4 (2013) 577

41. Andreyeva T, Puhl RM & Brownell KD. 'Changes in perceived weight discrimination among Americans, 1995–1996 through 2004–2006.' Obesity 16 (2008) 1129–1134

42. Sabin JA, Marini M & Nosek BA. 'Implicit and explicit anti-fat bias among a large sample of medical doctors by BMI, race/ethnicity and gender.' PLoS One 7 (2012) e48448

43. Puhl RM & Brownell KD. 'Confronting and coping with weight stigma: an investigation of overweight and obese adults.' Obesity 14 (2006) 1802–1815

44. Adams CH, Smith NJ, Wilbur DC & Grady KE. 'The relationship of obesity to the frequency of pelvic examinations: do physician and patient attitudes make a difference.' Women & Health 20 (1993) 45–57

45. Jenkins T. 'Jo attended for cervical smear. Nurse complained about fat making it difficult so said she should lose weight before she [. . .]' (2020). Retrieved from https://twitter.com/amnerisuk/status/1318906378153582594 (accessed Nov 2020)

46. Alberga AS, Edache IY, Forhan M & Russell-Mayhew S. 'Weight bias and health care utilization: a scoping review.' Primary Health Care Research & Development 20 (2019) e116

47. Phelan SM et al. 'The adverse effect of weight stigma on the well-being of medical students with overweight or obesity: Findings from a national survey.' Journal of General Internal Medicine 30 (2015) 1251–1258

48. Pearl RL & Puhl RM. 'Weight bias internalization and health: a systematic review.' Obesity Reviews 19 (2018) 1141–1163

49. Sikorski C, Luppa M, Luck T & Riedel-Heller SG. 'Weight stigma "gets under the skin" – evidence for an adapted psychological mediation framework: a systematic review.' Obesity 23 (2015) 266–276

50. Daly M, Robinson E & Sutin AR. 'Does Knowing Hurt? Perceiving Oneself as Overweight Predicts Future Physical Health and Well-Being.' Psychological Science 28 (2017) 872–881

51. Vadiveloo M & Mattei J. 'Perceived Weight Discrimination and 10-Year Risk of Allostatic Load Among US Adults.' Annals of Behavioral Medicine 51 (2017) 94–104

52. Pearl RL et al. 'Association between weight bias internalization and metabolic syndrome among treatment-seeking individuals with obesity.' Obesity 25 (2017) 317–322

53. Jackson SE, Beeken RJ & Wardle J. 'Perceived weight discrimination and changes in weight, waist circumference, and weight status.' Obesity 22 (2014) 2485–2488

54. Schvey NA, Puhl RM & Brownell KD. 'The impact of weight stigma on caloric consumption.' Obesity 19 (2011) 1957–1962

55. Jackson SE & Steptoe A. 'Association between perceived weight discrimination and physical activity: a population-based study among English middle-aged and older adults.' BMJ Open 7 (2017) e014592

56. Hilbert A et al. 'Risk factors across the eating disorders.' Psychiatry Research 220 (2014) 500–506

57. Shisslak CM, Crago M & Estes LS. 'The spectrum of eating disturbances.' International Journal of Eating Disorders 18 (1995) 209–219

58. Arcelus J, Mitchell AJ, Wales J & Nielsen S. 'Mortality rates in patients with anorexia nervosa and other eating disorders. A meta-analysis of 36 studies.' Archives Of General Psychiatry 68 (2011) 724–731

59. Raubenheimer D, Lee KP & Simpson SJ. 'Does Bertrand's rule apply to macronutrients.' Proceedings of the Royal Society B: Biological Sciences 272 (2005) 2429–2434

60. Weaver CM & Lappe JM. 'Robert Proulx Heaney, MD (1927–2016).' The Journal of Nutrition 147 (2017) 720–722

61. Fairweather D, Frisancho-Kiss S & Rose NR. 'Sex differences in autoimmune disease from a pathological perspective.' The American Journal of Pathology 173 (2008) 600–609

62. Maines RP. *The Technology of Orgasm* (JHU Press, 2001)

63. Chen EH et al. 'Gender disparity in analgesic treatment of emergency department patients with acute abdominal pain.' Academic Emergency Medicine 15 (2008) 414–418

64. Weisse CS, Sorum PC, Sanders KN & Syat BL. 'Do gender and race affect decisions about pain management.' Journal of General Internal Medicine 16 (2001) 211–217

65. Fardet A & Rock E. 'Perspective: Reductionist Nutrition Research Has Meaning Only within the Framework of Holistic and Ethical Thinking.' Advances in Nutrition 9 (2018) 655–670

66. Kalra B, Kalra S & Sharma JB. 'The inositols and polycystic ovary syndrome.' Indian Journal of Endocrinology and Metabolism 20 (2016) 720–724

67. Mach F et al. '2019 ESC/EAS Guidelines for the management of dyslipi-daemias: lipid modification to reduce cardiovascular risk.' European Heart Journal 41 (2020) 111–188

68. Banting W. *Letter on corpulence, addressed to the public* (Harrison, 1864)

69. Wadley L, Backwell L, d'Errico F & Sievers C. 'Cooked starchy rhizomes in Africa 170 thousand years ago.' Science 367 (2020) 87–91

70. BBC. 'The shocking amount of sugar hiding in your food – BBC' (2018). Retrieved from https://www.youtube.com/watch?v=eKQWFJmCWZE (accessed Aug 2020)

71. Wu X et al. 'Effects of the intestinal microbial metabolite butyrate on the development of colorectal cancer.' Journal of Cancer 9 (2018) 2510–2517

72. Stephen AM et al. 'Dietary fibre in Europe: current state of knowledge on definitions, sources, recommendations, intakes and relationships to health.' Nutrition Research Reviews 30 (2017) 149–190

73. Joye IJ. 'Dietary Fibre from Whole Grains and Their Benefits on Meta-bolic Health.' Nutrients 12 (2020) 3045

74. Hall H et al. 'Glucotypes reveal new patterns of glucose dysregulation.' PLoS Biology 16 (2018) e2005143

75. Raichle ME & Gusnard DA. 'Appraising the brain's energy budget.' Pro-ceedings of the National Academy of Sciences 99 (2002) 10237–10239

76. Lustig RH. 'Childhood obesity: behavioral aberration or biochemical drive? Reinterpreting the First Law of Thermodynamics.' Nature Clinical Practice Endocrinology & Metabolism 2 (2006) 447–458

77. Hall KD & Guo J. 'Obesity Energetics: Body Weight Regulation and the Effects of Diet Composition.' Gastroenterology 152 (2017) 1718–1727.e3

78. Hall KD et al. 'Calorie for Calorie, Dietary Fat Restriction Results in More Body Fat Loss than Carbohydrate Restriction in People with Obes-ity.' Cell Metabolism 22 (2015) 427–436

79. Horton TJ et al. 'Fat and carbohydrate overfeeding in humans: different effects on energy storage.' The American Journal of Clinical Nutrition 62 (1995) 19–29

80. Lammert O et al. 'Effects of isoenergetic overfeeding of either carbohy-drate or fat in young men.' British Journal of Nutrition 84 (2000) 233–245

81. McDevitt RM, Poppitt SD, Murgatroyd PR & Prentice AM. 'Macronu-trient disposal during controlled overfeeding with glucose, fructose, sucrose, or fat in lean and obese women.' The American Journal of Clin-ical Nutrition 72 (2000) 369–377

82. Guyenet S. 'Why the carbohydrate-insulin model of obesity is probably wrong: A supplementary reply to Ebbeling and Ludwig's JAMA article'

(2018). Retrieved from https://www.stephanguyenet.com/why-the-carbohydrate-insulin-model-of-obesity-is-probably-wrong-a-supplementary-reply-to-ebbeling-and-ludwigs-jama-article (accessed Apr 2020)

83. Organisation for Economic Co-operation and Development. *OECD Factbook 2015–2016: Economic, Environmental and Social Statistics* (OECD, 2016)

84. Oba S et al. 'Diet based on the Japanese Food Guide Spinning Top and subsequent mortality among men and women in a general Japanese population.' Journal of the American Dietetic Association 109 (2009) 1540–1547

85. Shan Z et al. 'Trends in Dietary Carbohydrate, Protein, and Fat Intake and Diet Quality Among US Adults, 1999–2016.' JAMA 322 (2019) 1178–1187

86. Hales CM, Carroll MD, Fryar CD & Ogden CL. 'Prevalence of obesity among adults and youth: United States, 2015–2016' (2017). Retrieved from https://www.cdc.gov/nchs/data/databriefs/db288.pdf (accessed June 2020)

87. Scientific Advisory Committee on Nutrition. 'Carbohydrates and Health' (2015). Retrieved from https://www.gov.uk/government/publications/sacn-carbohydrates-and-health-report (accessed June 2020)

88. Kreitzman SN, Coxon AY & Szaz KF. 'Glycogen storage: illusions of easy weight loss, excessive weight regain, and distortions in estimates of body composition.' The American Journal of Clinical Nutrition 56 (1992) 292–293

89. Te Morenga L, Mallard S & Mann J. 'Dietary sugars and body weight: systematic review and meta-analyses of randomised controlled trials and cohort studies.' BMJ 346 (2012) e7492

90. Hall KD et al. 'Ultra-Processed Diets Cause Excess Calorie Intake and Weight Gain: An Inpatient Randomized Controlled Trial of Ad Libitum Food Intake.' Cell Metabolism 30 (2019) 67–77.e3

91. Monteiro CA et al. 'The UN Decade of Nutrition, the NOVA food classification and the trouble with ultra-processing.' Public Health Nutrition 21 (2018) 5–17

92. Martínez Steele E, Raubenheimer D, Simpson SJ, Baraldi LG & Monteiro CA. 'Ultra-processed foods, protein leverage and energy intake in the USA.' Public Health Nutrition 21 (2018) 114–124

93. Fazzino TL, Rohde K & Sullivan DK. 'Hyper-Palatable Foods: Development of a Quantitative Definition and Application to the US Food System Database.' Obesity 27 (2019) 1761–1768

94. Morell P & Fiszman S. 'Revisiting the role of protein-induced satiation and satiety.' Food Hydrocolloids 68 (2017) 199–210

95. Keller A & Bucher Della Torre S. 'Sugar-Sweetened Beverages and Obesity among Children and Adolescents: A Review of Systematic Literature Reviews.' Childhood Obesity 11 (2015) 338–346

96. Kaiser KA, Shikany JM, Keating KD & Allison DB. 'Will reducing sugar-sweetened beverage consumption reduce obesity? Evidence supporting conjecture is strong, but evidence when testing effect is weak.' Obesity Reviews 14 (2013) 620–633

97. Malik VS, Pan A, Willett WC & Hu FB. 'Sugar-sweetened beverages and weight gain in children and adults: a systematic review and meta-analysis.' The American Journal of Clinical Nutrition 98 (2013) 1084–1102

98. Pan A & Hu FB. 'Effects of carbohydrates on satiety: differences between liquid and solid food.' Current Opinion in Clinical Nutrition & Metabolic Care 14 (2011) 385–390

99. Almiron-Roig E et al. 'Factors that determine energy compensation: a systematic review of preload studies.' Nutrition Reviews 71 (2013) 458–473

100. St-Onge MP et al. 'Added thermogenic and satiety effects of a mixed nutrient vs a sugar-only beverage.' International Journal of Obesity and Related Metabolic Disorders 28 (2004) 248–253

101. DellaValle DM, Roe LS & Rolls BJ. 'Does the consumption of caloric and non-caloric beverages with a meal affect energy intake.' Appetite 44 (2005) 187–193

102. Yang Q et al. 'Added sugar intake and cardiovascular diseases mortality among US adults.' JAMA Internal Medicine 174 (2014) 516–524

103. Department for Environment, Food and Rural Affairs. 'National Food Survey' (2000). Retrieved from https://data.gov.uk/dataset/5c1a7a5d-4dd5-4b1b-84f2-3ba8883a07ca/family-food-open-data (accessed July 2020)

104. Department for Environment, Food and Rural Affairs. 'Expenditure and Food Survey' (2007). Retrieved from https://www.gov.uk/government/statistical-data-sets/family-food-datasets (accessed July 2020)

105. Department for Environment, Food and Rural Affairs. 'Living Costs and Food Survey' (2019). Retrieved from https://www.gov.uk/government/statistical-data-sets/family-food-datasets (accessed July 2020)

106. Mansoor N, Vinknes KJ, Veierød MB & Retterstøl K. 'Effects of low-carbohydrate diets v. low-fat diets on body weight and cardiovascular risk factors: a meta-analysis of randomised controlled trials.' British Journal of Nutrition 115 (2016) 466–479

107. Nazare J-A et al. 'Ethnic influences on the relations between abdominal subcutaneous and visceral adiposity, liver fat, and cardiometabolic risk profile: the International Study of Prediction of Intra-Abdominal Adiposity and Its Relationship With Cardiometabolic Risk/Intra-Abdominal Adiposity.' The American Journal of Clinical Nutrition 96 (2012) 714–726

108. Wolever TM. 'Dietary carbohydrates and insulin action in humans.' British Journal of Nutrition 83 (2000) S97–102

109. Macdonald IA. 'A review of recent evidence relating to sugars, insulin resistance and diabetes.' European Journal of Nutrition 55 (2016) 17–23

110. Hodson L, Rosqvist F & Parry SA. 'The influence of dietary fatty acids on liver fat content and metabolism – ERRATUM.' Proceedings of the Nutrition Society 78 (2019) 473

111. Soechtig S, Couric K & David L. 'FED UP – Official Trailer' (2014). Retrieved from https://www.youtube.com/watch?v=aCUbvOwwfWM (accessed July 2020)

112. DiNicolantonio JJ, O'Keefe JH & Wilson WL. 'Sugar addiction: is it real? A narrative review.' British Journal of Sports Medicine 52 (2018) 910–913

113. Avena NM, Rada P & Hoebel BG. 'Evidence for sugar addiction: behavioral and neurochemical effects of intermittent, excessive sugar intake.' Neuroscience & Biobehavioral Reviews 32 (2008) 20–39

114. Westwater ML, Fletcher PC & Ziauddeen H. 'Sugar addiction: the state of the science.' European Journal of Nutrition 55 (2016) 55–69

115. Avena NM, Rada P & Hoebel BG. 'Underweight rats have enhanced dopamine release and blunted acetylcholine response in the nucleus accumbens while bingeing on sucrose.' Neuroscience 156 (2008) 865–871

116. Stice E, Davis K, Miller NP & Marti CN. 'Fasting increases risk for onset of binge eating and bulimic pathology: a 5-year prospective study.' Journal of Abnormal Psychology 117 (2008) 941–946

117. Yanovski S. 'Sugar and fat: cravings and aversions.' Journal of Nutrition 133 (2003) 835S–837S

118. Davis N. 'Is sugar really as addictive as cocaine? Scientists row over effect on body and brain' (2017). Retrieved from https://www.theguardian.com/society/2017/aug/25/is-sugar-really-as-addictive-as-cocaine-scientists-row-over-effect-on-body-and-brain (accessed July 2020)

119. Tandel KR. 'Sugar substitutes: Health controversy over perceived benefits.' Journal of Pharmacology & Pharmacotherapeutics 2 (2011) 236–243

120. Ruiz-Ojeda FJ, Plaza-Díaz J, Sáez-Lara MJ & Gil A. 'Effects of Sweeteners on the Gut Microbiota: A Review of Experimental Studies and Clinical Trials.' Advances in Nutrition 10 (2019) S31–S48

121. Renwick AG & Molinary SV. 'Sweet-taste receptors, low-energy sweeteners, glucose absorption and insulin release.' British Journal of Nutrition 104 (2010) 1415–1420

122. Tucker RM & Tan SY. 'Do non-nutritive sweeteners influence acute glucose homeostasis in humans? A systematic review.' Physiology & Behavior 182 (2017) 17–26

123. Schiffman SS et al. 'Aspartame and susceptibility to headache.' New England Journal of Medicine 317 (1987) 1181–1185

124. Thannhauser SJ & Magendantz H. 'The different clinical groups of xanthomatous diseases: a clinical physiological study of 22 cases.' Annals of Internal Medicine 11 (1938) 1662–1746

125. Castelli WP, Anderson K, Wilson PW & Levy D. 'Lipids and risk of coronary heart disease. The Framingham Study.' Annals of Epidemiology 2 (1992) 23–28

126. Sharrett AR et al. 'Coronary heart disease prediction from lipoprotein cholesterol levels, triglycerides, lipoprotein(a), apolipoproteins A-I and B, and HDL density subfractions: The Atherosclerosis Risk in Communities (ARIC) Study.' Circulation 104 (2001) 1108–1113

127. Silverman MG et al. 'Association Between Lowering LDL-C and Cardiovascular Risk Reduction Among Different Therapeutic Interventions: A Systematic Review and Meta-analysis.' JAMA 316 (2016) 1289–1297

128. Cholesterol Treatment Trialists' Collaboration. 'Efficacy and safety of statin therapy in older people: a meta-analysis of individual participant data from 28 randomised controlled trials.' The Lancet 393 (2019) 407–415

129. Keene D, Price C, Shun-Shin MJ & Francis DP. 'Effect on cardiovascular risk of high density lipoprotein targeted drug treatments niacin, fibrates, and CETP inhibitors: meta-analysis of randomised controlled trials including 117,411 patients.' BMJ 349 (2014) g4379

130. Millán J et al. 'Lipoprotein ratios: physiological significance and clinical usefulness in cardiovascular prevention.' Vascular Health and Risk Management 5 (2009) 757

131. Prospective Studies Collaboration. 'Blood cholesterol and vascular mortality by age, sex, and blood pressure: a meta-analysis of individual data from 61 prospective studies with 55 000 vascular deaths.' The Lancet 370 (2007) 1829–1839

132. Mozaffarian D, Katan MB, Ascherio A, Stampfer MJ & Willett WC. 'Trans fatty acids and cardiovascular disease.' New England Journal of Medicine 354 (2006) 1601–1613

133. Clifton PM & Keogh JB. 'A systematic review of the effect of dietary saturated and polyunsaturated fat on heart disease.' Nutrition, Metabolism & Cardiovascular Diseases 27 (2017) 1060–1080

134. Hooper L et al. 'Reduction in saturated fat intake for cardiovascular disease.' Cochrane Database of Systematic Reviews (2020)

135. NHS. 'Fat: the facts' (2020). Retrieved from https://www.nhs.uk/live-well/eat-well/different-fats-nutrition (accessed Dec 2020)

136. Thorning TK et al. 'Whole dairy matrix or single nutrients in assessment of health effects: current evidence and knowledge gaps.' The American Journal of Clinical Nutrition 105 (2017) 1033–1045

137. Hollænder PL, Ross AB & Kristensen M. 'Whole-grain and blood lipid changes in apparently healthy adults: a systematic review and meta-analysis of randomized controlled studies.' The American Journal of Clinical Nutrition 102 (2015) 556–572

138. Threapleton DE et al. 'Dietary fibre intake and risk of cardiovascular disease: systematic review and meta-analysis.' BMJ 347 (2013) f6879

139. Borén J et al. 'Low-density lipoproteins cause atherosclerotic cardiovascular disease: pathophysiological, genetic, and therapeutic insights: a consensus statement from the European Atherosclerosis Society Consensus Panel.' European Heart Journal 41 (2020) 2313–2330

140. Sacks FM et al. 'Dietary Fats and Cardiovascular Disease: A Presidential Advisory From the American Heart Association.' Circulation 136 (2017) e1–e23

141. Dagenais GR et al. 'Variations in common diseases, hospital admissions, and deaths in middle-aged adults in 21 countries from five continents (PURE): a prospective cohort study.' The Lancet 395 (2020) 785–794

142. Martinez-Gonzalez MA & Martin-Calvo N. 'Mediterranean diet and life expectancy; beyond olive oil, fruits, and vegetables.' Current Opinion in Clinical Nutrition & Metabolic Care 19 (2016) 401–407

143. British Dietetic Association. 'Top 5 worst celeb diets to avoid in 2018' (2017). Retrieved from https://www.bda.uk.com/resource/top-5-worst-celeb-diets-to-avoid-in-2018.html (accessed Nov 2020)

144. Matthews A et al. 'Impact of statin related media coverage on use of statins: interrupted time series analysis with UK primary care data.' BMJ 353 (2016) i3283

145. Nissen SE et al. 'Effect of very high-intensity statin therapy on regression of coronary atherosclerosis: the ASTEROID trial.' JAMA 295 (2006) 1556–1565

146. Mann GV, Pearson G, Gordon T & Dawber TR. 'Diet and cardiovascular disease in the Framingham study. I. Measurement of dietary intake.' The American Journal of Clinical Nutrition 11 (1962) 200–225

147. Lecerf J-M & De Lorgeril M. 'Dietary cholesterol: from physiology to cardiovascular risk.' British Journal of Nutrition 106 (2011) 6–14

148. Katan MB & Beynen AC. 'Characteristics of human hypo-and hyperresponders to dietary cholesterol.' American Journal of Public Health 125 (1987) 387–399

149. Blesso CN & Fernandez ML. 'Dietary cholesterol, serum lipids, and heart disease: are eggs working for or against you.' Nutrients 10 (2018) 426

150. Herron KL et al. 'Men classified as hypo-or hyperresponders to dietary cholesterol feeding exhibit differences in lipoprotein metabolism.' The Journal of Nutrition 133 (2003) 1036–1042

151. Herron KL, Lofgren IE, Sharman M, Volek JS & Fernandez ML. 'High intake of cholesterol results in less atherogenic low-density lipoprotein particles in men and women independent of response classification.' Metabolism 53 (2004) 823–830

152. Melough MM, Chung SJ, Fernandez ML & Chun OK. 'Association of eggs with dietary nutrient adequacy and cardiovascular risk factors in US adults.' Public Health Nutrition 22 (2019) 2033–2042

153. Bellanger N et al. 'Atheroprotective reverse cholesterol transport pathway is defective in familial hypercholesterolemia.' Arteriosclerosis, thrombosis, and vascular biology 31 (2011) 1675–1681

154. Santos S, Oliveira A & Lopes C. 'Systematic review of saturated fatty acids on inflammation and circulating levels of adipokines.' Nutrition Research 33 (2013) 687–695

155. Drouin-Chartier J-P et al. 'Systematic review of the association between dairy product consumption and risk of cardiovascular-related clinical outcomes.' Advances in Nutrition 7 (2016) 1026–1040

156. Mozaffarian D. 'Dairy Foods, Obesity, and Metabolic Health: The Role of the Food Matrix Compared with Single Nutrients.' Advances in Nutrition 10 (2019) 917S-923S

157. Bordoni A et al. 'Dairy products and inflammation: A review of the clinical evidence.' Critical Reviews in Food Science and Nutrition 57 (2017) 2497–2525

158. Spence JD, Jenkins DJ & Davignon J. 'Egg yolk consumption and carotid plaque.' Atherosclerosis 224 (2012) 469–473

159. Magriplis E et al. 'Frequency and Quantity of Egg Intake Is Not Associated with Dyslipidemia: The Hellenic National Nutrition and Health Survey (HNNHS).' Nutrients 11 (2019) 1105

160. Derbyshire E. 'Brain Health across the lifespan: A systematic review on the role of omega-3 fatty acid supplements.' Nutrients 10 (2018) 1094

161. Abdelhamid AS et al. 'Omega-3 fatty acids for the primary and secondary prevention of cardiovascular disease.' Cochrane Database of Systematic Reviews (2020)

162. Skulas-Ray AC et al. 'Omega-3 fatty acids for the management of hypertriglyceridemia: a science advisory from the American Heart Association.' Circulation 140 (2019) e673–e691

163. Lin L et al. 'Evidence of health benefits of canola oil.' Nutrition Reviews 71 (2013) 370–385

164. Harris WS et al. 'Omega-6 fatty acids and risk for cardiovascular disease: a science advisory from the American Heart Association Nutrition Subcommittee of the Council on Nutrition, Physical Activity, and Metabolism;

Council on Cardiovascular Nursing; and Council on Epidemiology and Prevention.' Circulation 119 (2009) 902–907

165. Marklund M et al. 'Biomarkers of dietary omega-6 fatty acids and incident cardiovascular disease and mortality: an individual-level pooled analysis of 30 cohort studies.' Circulation 139 (2019) 2422–2436

166. Stanley JC et al. 'UK Food Standards Agency Workshop Report: the effects of the dietary n-6: n-3 fatty acid ratio on cardiovascular health.' British Journal of Nutrition 98 (2007) 1305–1310

167. Johnson GH & Fritsche K. 'Effect of dietary linoleic acid on markers of inflammation in healthy persons: a systematic review of randomized controlled trials.' Journal of the Academy of Nutrition and Dietetics 112 (2012) 1029–1041

168. Rett BS & Whelan J. 'Increasing dietary linoleic acid does not increase tissue arachidonic acid content in adults consuming Western-type diets: a systematic review.' Nutrition & Metabolism 8 (2011) 36

169. Neelakantan N, Seah JYH & van Dam RM. 'The Effect of Coconut Oil Consumption on Cardiovascular Risk Factors: A Systematic Review and Meta-Analysis of Clinical Trials.' Circulation 141 (2020) 803–814

170. Gaforio JJ et al. 'Virgin olive oil and health: summary of the III international conference on virgin olive oil and health consensus report, JAEN (Spain) 2018.' Nutrients 11 (2019) 2039

171. Select Committee on Nutrition and Human Needs. *Dietary goals for the United States* (U.S. Government Printing Office, 1977)

172. National Advisory Committee on Nutrition Education. *A Discussion Paper on Proposals for Nutritional Guidelines for Health Education in Britain* (NACNE, 1983)

173. Krebs-Smith SM, Guenther PM, Subar AF, Kirkpatrick SI & Dodd KW. 'Americans do not meet federal dietary recommendations.' Journal of Nutrition 140 (2010) 1832–1838

174. Estruch R et al. 'Primary prevention of cardiovascular disease with a Mediterranean diet supplemented with extra-virgin olive oil or nuts.' New England Journal of Medicine 378 (2018) e34

175. Sprague RG. 'Russell Morse Wilder, Sr. 1885–1959.' Diabetes 9 (1960) 419–420

176. D'Andrea Meira I et al. 'Ketogenic Diet and Epilepsy: What We Know So Far.' Frontiers in Neuroscience 13 (2019) 5

177. Liu H et al. 'Ketogenic diet for treatment of intractable epilepsy in adults: A meta-analysis of observational studies.' Epilepsia Open 3 (2018) 9–17

178. Pugliese MT, Lifshitz F, Grad G, Fort P & Marks-Katz M. 'Fear of obesity. A cause of short stature and delayed puberty.' New England Journal of Medicine 309 (1983) 513–518

179. Ballaban-Gil K et al. 'Complications of the ketogenic diet.' Epilepsia 39 (1998) 744–748

180. Blanco JC, Khatri A, Kifayat A, Cho R & Aronow WS. 'Starvation Ketoacidosis due to the Ketogenic Diet and Prolonged Fasting–A Possibly Dangerous Diet Trend.' The American Journal of Case Reports 20 (2019) 1728

181. von Geijer L & Ekelund M. 'Ketoacidosis associated with low-carbohydrate diet in a non-diabetic lactating woman: a case report.' Journal of Medical Case Reports 9 (2015) 224

182. Zilberter T & Zilberter Y. 'Ketogenic ratio determines metabolic effects of macronutrients and prevents interpretive bias.' Frontiers in Nutrition 5 (2018)

183. Tzur A, Nijholt R, Sparangna V & Ritson A. 'Adhering to the Ketogenic Diet – Is it Easy or Hard? (Research Review)' (2018). Retrieved from https://sci-fit.net/adhere-ketogenic-diet (accessed Aug 2020)

184. Ting R, Dugré N, Allan GM & Lindblad AJ. 'Ketogenic diet for weight loss.' Canadian Family Physician 64 (2018) 906

185. Hall KD et al. 'Energy expenditure and body composition changes after an isocaloric ketogenic diet in overweight and obese men.' The American Journal of Clinical Nutrition 104 (2016) 324–333

186. Lemstra M, Bird Y, Nwankwo C, Rogers M & Moraros J. 'Weight loss intervention adherence and factors promoting adherence: a meta-analysis.' Patient Preference and Adherence 10 (2016) 1547

187. Ye F, Li X-J, Jiang W-L, Sun H-B & Liu J. 'Efficacy of and patient compliance with a ketogenic diet in adults with intractable epilepsy: a meta-analysis.' Journal of Clinical Neurology 11 (2015) 26–31

188. Zupec-Kania B. 'Micronutrient content of an optimally selected ketogenic diet.' Journal of the American Dietetic Association 103 (2003) 8–9

189. Johnston CS et al. 'Ketogenic low-carbohydrate diets have no metabolic advantage over nonketogenic low-carbohydrate diets.' The American Journal of Clinical Nutrition 83 (2006) 1055–1061

190. Snorgaard O, Poulsen GM, Andersen HK & Astrup A. 'Systematic review and meta-analysis of dietary carbohydrate restriction in patients with type 2 diabetes.' BMJ Open Diabetes Research and Care 5 (2017)

191. Lean MEJ et al. 'Primary care-led weight management for remission of type 2 diabetes (DiRECT): an open-label, cluster-randomised trial.' The Lancet 391 (2018) 541–551

192. Hemalatha R, Ramalaxmi BA, Swetha E, Balakrishna N & Mastromarino P. 'Evaluation of vaginal pH for detection of bacterial vaginosis.' The Indian Journal of Medical Research 138 (2013) 354

193. Bostock E, Kirkby KC & Taylor BVM. 'The current status of the ketogenic diet in psychiatry.' Frontiers in Psychiatry 8 (2017) 43

194. Stubbs BJ et al. 'On the metabolism of exogenous ketones in humans.' Frontiers in Physiology 8 (2017) 848

195. Schübel R et al. 'Effects of intermittent and continuous calorie restriction on body weight and metabolism over 50 wk: A randomized controlled trial.' The American Journal of Clinical Nutrition 108 (2018) 933–945

196. Shang L et al. 'Nutrient starvation elicits an acute autophagic response mediated by Ulk1 dephosphorylation and its subsequent dissociation from AMPK.' Proceedings of the National Academy of Sciences 108 (2011) 4788–4793

197. Yoshii SR & Mizushima N. 'Monitoring and Measuring Autophagy.' International Journal of Molecular Sciences 18 (2017) 1865

198. Satija A et al. 'Healthful and Unhealthful Plant-Based Diets and the Risk of Coronary Heart Disease in U.S. Adults.' Journal of the American College of Cardiology 70 (2017) 411–422

199. Song M et al. 'Association of Animal and Plant Protein Intake With All-Cause and Cause-Specific Mortality.' JAMA Internal Medicine 176 (2016) 1453–1463

200. Tong TYN et al. 'Risks of ischaemic heart disease and stroke in meat eaters, fish eaters, and vegetarians over 18 years of follow-up: results from the prospective EPIC-Oxford study.' bmj 366 (2019) l4897

201. PETA. 'Cow's Milk: A Cruel and Unhealthy Product' (2013). Retrieved from https://www.peta.org/issues/animals-used-for-food/animals-used-food-factsheets/cows-milk-cruel-unhealthy-product (accessed Aug 2020)

202. Alexander RT, Cordat E, Chambrey R, Dimke H & Eladari D. 'Acidosis and urinary calcium excretion: insights from genetic disorders.' Journal of the American Society of Nephrology 27 (2016) 3511–3520

203. Kerstetter JE, Kenny AM & Insogna KL. 'Dietary protein and skeletal health: a review of recent human research.' Current Opinion in Lipidology 22 (2011) 16

204. Chan GM, Hoffman K & McMurry M. 'Effects of dairy products on bone and body composition in pubertal girls.' The Journal of Pediatrics 126 (1995) 551–556

205. Baran D et al. 'Dietary modification with dairy products for preventing vertebral bone loss in premenopausal women: a three-year prospective study.' The Journal of Clinical Endocrinology and Metabolism 70 (1990) 264–270

206. Appleby P, Roddam A, Allen N & Key T. 'Comparative fracture risk in vegetarians and nonvegetarians in EPIC-Oxford.' European Journal of Clinical Nutrition 61 (2007) 1400–1406

207. Ornish D et al. 'Can lifestyle changes reverse coronary heart disease? The Lifestyle Heart Trial.' The Lancet 336 (1990) 129–133

208. Tawakol A et al. 'Relation between resting amygdalar activity and cardio-vascular events: a longitudinal and cohort study.' The Lancet 389 (2017) 834–845

209. Hong MK et al. 'Limitations of angiography for analyzing coronary ath-erosclerosis progression or regression.' Annals of Internal Medicine 121 (1994) 348–354

210. Berry C et al. 'Comparison of intravascular ultrasound and quantitative coronary angiography for the assessment of coronary artery disease pro-gression.' Circulation 115 (2007) 1851–1857

211. Devries MC et al. 'Changes in kidney function do not differ between healthy adults consuming higher-compared with lower-or normal-protein diets: a systematic review and meta-analysis.' The Journal of Nutrition 148 (2018) 1760–1775

212. Rhee CM, Ahmadi S, Kovesdy CP & Kalantar-Zadeh K. 'Low-protein diet for conservative management of chronic kidney disease: a systematic review and meta-analysis of controlled trials.' Journal of Cachexia, Sarco-penia and Muscle 9 (2018) 235–245

213. Ravel VA et al. 'Low protein nitrogen appearance as a surrogate of low dietary protein intake is associated with higher all-cause mortality in maintenance hemodialysis patients.' The Journal of Nutrition 143 (2013) 1084–1092

214. Agency for Healthcare Research and Quality. 'Healthy Men: Learn the Facts' (2012). Retrieved from https://archive.ahrq.gov/patients-consumers/patient-involvement/healthy-men/index.html (accessed Sept 2020)

215. Deng J. 'Goop, Inc. Settles Consumer Protection Lawsuit Over Three Wellness Products' (2018). Retrieved from https://www.sccgov.org/sites/da/newsroom/newsreleases/Pages/NRA2018/Goop.aspx (accessed Dec 2020)

216. Gunter J. 'Dear Gwyneth Paltrow, I'm a GYN and your vaginal jade eggs are a bad idea' (2017). Retrieved from https://drjengunter.com/2017/01/17/dear-gwyneth-paltrow-im-a-gyn-and-your-vaginal-jade-eggs-are-a-bad-idea (accessed Dec 2020)

217. Kam-Hansen S et al. 'Altered placebo and drug labeling changes the out-come of episodic migraine attacks.' Science Translational Medicine 6 (2014) 218ra5

218. Saladino P. 'How You've Been Misled About Red Meat Causing Diabetes and Heart Disease, With Ex-Vegan, Jon Venus' (2020). Retrieved from https://carnivoremd.com/how-youve-been-misled-about-red-meat-causing-diabetes-and-heart-disease-with-ex-vegan-jon-venus (accessed Dec 2020)

219. Saladino P. 'Controversial Thoughts: Carnivore Diet for Beginners' (2020). Retrieved from https://www.youtube.com/watch?v=8T6N9Y9VDe0 (accessed Nov 2020)

220. Saladino P. *The Carnivore Code* (Houghton Mifflin Harcourt, 2020)

221. Peterson M. 'Twitter Profile' (2020). Retrieved from https://twitter.com/MikhailaAleksis (accessed Sept 2020)

222. Peterson M. 'About Me' (2020). Retrieved from https://mikhailapeterson.com/about (accessed Sept 2020)

223. Bowles N. 'Jordan Peterson, Custodian of the Patriarchy' (2018). Retrieved from https://www.nytimes.com/2018/05/18/style/jordan-peterson-12-rules-for-life.html (accessed Nov 2020)

224. JRE Clips. 'Joe Rogan – Jordan Peterson's Carnivore Diet Cured His Depression?' (2018). Retrieved from https://www.youtube.com/watch?v=HLF29w6YqXs (accessed July 2020)

225. Dunner D et al. 'Preventing recurrent depression: long-term treatment for major depressive disorder.' Primary Care Companion to The Journal of Clinical Psychiatry 9 (2007) 214–223

226. Preston BD, Albertson TM & Herr AJ. 'DNA replication fidelity and cancer.' Seminars in Cancer Biology 20 (2010) 281–293

227. Cancer Research UK. 'Cancer survival statistics for all cancers combined' (2014). Retrieved from https://www.cancerresearchuk.org/health-professional/cancer-statistics/survival/all-cancers-combined (accessed July 2020)

228. Huebner J et al. 'Counseling patients on cancer diets: a review of the literature and recommendations for clinical practice.' Anticancer Research 34 (2014) 39–48

229. Buckner CA, Lafrenie RM, Dénommée JA, Caswell JM & Want DA. 'Complementary and alternative medicine use in patients before and after a cancer diagnosis.' Current Oncology 25 (2018) e275

230. Johnson SB, Park HS, Gross CP & Yu JB. 'Use of alternative medicine for cancer and its impact on survival.' Journal of the National Cancer Institute 110 (2018) 121–124

231. Ho PJ et al. 'Impact of delayed treatment in women diagnosed with breast cancer: A population-based study.' Cancer Medicine 9 (2020) 2435–2444

232. United Nations, Department of Economic and Social Affairs, Population Division. 'World Population Prospects 2019, Volume I: Comprehensive Tables' (2019). Retrieved from https://population.un.org/wpp/Publications/ (accessed Oct 2020)

233. Roser M & Ritchie H. 'Cancer' (2015). Retrieved from https://ourworldindata.org/cancer (accessed July 2020)

234. Dellavedova T. 'Prostatic specific antigen. From its early days until becoming a prostate cancer biomarker.' Archivos Españoles de Urología 69 (2016) 19–23

235. American Cancer Society. 'Cancer Facts & Figures 2020' (2020). Retrieved from https://www.cancer.org/research/cancer-facts-statistics/all-cancer-facts-figures/cancer-facts-figures-2020 (accessed July 2020)

236. Sasieni PD, Shelton J, Ormiston-Smith N, Thomson CS & Silcocks PB. 'What is the lifetime risk of developing cancer?: the effect of adjusting for multiple primaries.' British Journal of Cancer 105 (2011) 460–465

237. Cancer Research UK. 'Does obesity cause cancer?' (2018). Retrieved from https://www.cancerresearchuk.org/about-cancer/causes-of-cancer/obesity-weight-and-cancer/does-obesity-cause-cancer (accessed July 2020)

238. Afzal S, Tybjærg-Hansen A, Jensen GB & Nordestgaard BG. 'Change in body mass index associated with lowest mortality in Denmark, 1976–2013.' JAMA 315 (2016) 1989–1996

239. Puhl RM, Andreyeva T & Brownell KD. 'Perceptions of weight discrimination: prevalence and comparison to race and gender discrimination in America.' International journal of obesity 32 (2008) 992–1000

240. Kyrgiou M et al. 'Adiposity and cancer at major anatomical sites: umbrella review of the literature.' BMJ 356 (2017) j477

241. Yang X-J, Jiang H-M, Hou X-H & Song J. 'Anxiety and depression in patients with gastroesophageal reflux disease and their effect on quality of life.' World Journal of Gastroenterology 21 (2015) 4302

242. Song EM, Jung H-K & Jung JM. 'The association between reflux esophagitis and psychosocial stress.' Digestive Diseases and Sciences 58 (2013) 471–477

243. Galéra C et al. 'Stress, attention deficit hyperactivity disorder (ADHD) symptoms and tobacco smoking: The i-Share study.' European Psychiatry 45 (2017) 221–226

244. Slopen N et al. 'Psychosocial stress and cigarette smoking persistence, cessation, and relapse over 9–10 years: a prospective study of middle-aged adults in the United States.' Cancer Causes & Control 24 (2013) 1849–1863

245. Keyes KM, Hatzenbuehler ML, Grant BF & Hasin DS. 'Stress and alcohol: Epidemiologic evidence.' Alcohol Research: Current Reviews 34 (2012) 391–400

246. Wu Y & Berry DC. 'Impact of weight stigma on physiological and psychological health outcomes for overweight and obese adults: a systematic review.' Journal of Advanced Nursing 74 (2018) 1030–1042

247. NHS Digital. 'National Child Measurement Programme, England 2018/19 School Year [NS]' (2019). Retrieved from https://digital.nhs.uk/data-and-information/publications/statistical/national-child-measurement-programme/2018-19-school-year/deprivation (accessed July 2020)

248. Almeida DM, Neupert SD, Banks SR & Serido J. 'Do daily stress processes account for socioeconomic health disparities.' The Journals of Gerontology Series B 60 (2005) S34–S39

249. Kubo A, Corley DA, Jensen CD & Kaur R. 'Dietary factors and the risks of oesophageal adenocarcinoma and Barrett's oesophagus.' Nutrition Research Reviews 23 (2010) 230–246

250. Brown KF et al. 'The fraction of cancer attributable to modifiable risk factors in England, Wales, Scotland, Northern Ireland, and the United Kingdom in 2015.' British Journal of Cancer 118 (2018) 1130–1141

251. Schoemaker MJ et al. 'Association of body mass index and age with subsequent breast cancer risk in premenopausal women.' JAMA oncology 4 (2018) e181771–e181771

252. Carr D & Friedman MA. 'Is obesity stigmatizing? Body weight, perceived discrimination, and psychological well-being in the United States.' Journal of Health and Social Behavior 46 (2005) 244–259

253. Hebl MR, Xu J & Mason MF. 'Weighing the care: patients' perceptions of physician care as a function of gender and weight.' International Journal of Obesity and Related Metabolic Disorders 27 (2003) 269–275

254. Rafiee P et al. 'Sugar Sweetened Beverages and Cancer: a Brief Review.' Current Topics in Nutraceutical Research 15 (2017)

255. Miles FL, Neuhouser ML & Zhang Z-F. 'Concentrated sugars and incidence of prostate cancer in a prospective cohort.' British Journal of Nutrition 120 (2018) 703–710

256. Romanos-Nanclares A et al. 'Sugar-sweetened beverage consumption and incidence of breast cancer: the Seguimiento Universidad de Navarra (SUN) Project.' European Journal of Nutrition 58 (2019) 2875–2886

257. Chazelas E et al. 'Sugary drink consumption and risk of cancer: results from NutriNet-Santé prospective cohort.' BMJ 366 (2019) l2408

258. Bassett JK, Milne RL, English DR, Giles GG & Hodge AM. 'Consumption of sugar-sweetened and artificially sweetened soft drinks and risk of cancers not related to obesity.' International Journal of Cancer 146 (2020) 3329–3334

259. Shingler E et al. 'Dietary restriction during the treatment of cancer: results of a systematic scoping review.' BMC cancer 19 (2019) 811

260. Erickson N, Boscheri A, Linke B & Huebner JJMO. 'Systematic review: isocaloric ketogenic dietary regimes for cancer patients.' Medical Oncology 34 (2017) 72

261. Sremanakova J, Sowerbutts AM & Burden S. 'A systematic review of the use of ketogenic diets in adult patients with cancer.' Journal of Human Nutrition and Dietetics 31 (2018) 793–802

262. Warburg O. 'The metabolism of carcinoma cells.' The Journal of Cancer Research 9 (1925) 148–163

263. Cardone RA, Casavola V & Reshkin SJ. 'The role of disturbed pH dynamics and the Na+/H+ exchanger in metastasis.' Nature Reviews Cancer 5 (2005) 786–795

264. Fenton TR & Huang T. 'Systematic review of the association between dietary acid load, alkaline water and cancer.' BMJ Open 6 (2016) e010438

265. Hendrix MJ, Seftor EA, Seftor RE & Fidler IJ. 'A simple quantitative assay for studying the invasive potential of high and low human metastatic variants.' Cancer Letters 38 (1987) 137–147

266. Koufman JA & Johnston N. 'Potential benefits of pH 8.8 alkaline drinking water as an adjunct in the treatment of reflux disease.' Annals of Otology, Rhinology, and Laryngology 121 (2012) 431–434

267. Kozisek F. *Nutrients in Drinking Water* (World Health Organization, 2005)

268. Haighton L, Roberts A, Walters B & Lynch B. 'Systematic review and evaluation of aspartame carcinogenicity bioassays using quality criteria.' Regulatory Toxicology and Pharmacology 103 (2019) 332–344

269. Boyle P, Koechlin A & Autier P. 'Sweetened carbonated beverage consumption and cancer risk: meta-analysis and review.' European Journal of Cancer Prevention 23 (2014) 481–490

270. Mishra A, Ahmed K, Froghi S & Dasgupta P. 'Systematic review of the relationship between artificial sweetener consumption and cancer in humans: analysis of 599,741 participants.' International Journal of Clinical Practice 69 (2015) 1418–1426

271. Cancer Research UK. 'Do artificial sweeteners cause cancer?' (2019). Retrievedfromhttps://www.cancerresearchuk.org/about-cancer/causes-of-cancer/cancer-controversies/do-artificial-sweeteners-cause-cancer (accessed July 2020)

272. Cattaruzza MS & West R. 'Why do doctors and medical students smoke when they must know how harmful it is.' European Journal of Public Health 23 (2013) 188–189

273. Chan DS et al. 'Red and processed meat and colorectal cancer incidence: meta-analysis of prospective studies.' PLoS One 6 (2011) e20456

274. Etemadi A et al. 'Mortality from different causes associated with meat, heme iron, nitrates, and nitrites in the NIH-AARP Diet and Health Study: population based cohort study.' BMJ 357 (2017) j1957

275. McDonald JA, Goyal A & Terry MB. 'Alcohol intake and breast cancer risk: weighing the overall evidence.' Current Breast Cancer Reports 5 (2013) 208–221

276. MacMahon B et al. 'Age at first birth and breast cancer risk.' Bulletin of the World Health Organization 43 (1970) 209

277. Weroha SJ & Haluska P. 'The insulin-like growth factor system in cancer.' Endocrinology and Metabolism Clinics of North America 41 (2012) 335–50, vi

278. Collier RJ & Bauman DE. 'Update on human health concerns of recombinant bovine somatotropin use in dairy cows.' Journal of Animal Science 92 (2014) 1800–1807

279. Mero A et al. 'IGF-I, IgA, and IgG responses to bovine colostrum supplementation during training.' Journal of Applied Physiology 93 (2002) 732–739

280. Travis RC & Key TJ. 'Oestrogen exposure and breast cancer risk.' Breast Cancer Research 5 (2003) 239

281. Macrina AL, Ott TL, Roberts RF & Kensinger RS. 'Estrone and estrone sulfate concentrations in milk and milk fractions.' Journal of the Academy of Nutrition and Dietetics 112 (2012) 1088–1093

282. Larsson SC, Crippa A, Orsini N, Wolk A & Michaëlsson K. 'Milk consumption and mortality from all causes, cardiovascular disease, and cancer: a systematic review and meta-analysis.' Nutrients 7 (2015) 7749–7763

283. Ma J et al. 'Milk intake, circulating levels of insulin-like growth factor-I, and risk of colorectal cancer in men.' Journal of the National Cancer Institute 93 (2001) 1330–1336

284. Mukhopadhyay S, Panda PK, Sinha N, Das DN & Bhutia SK. 'Autophagy and apoptosis: where do they meet.' Apoptosis 19 (2014) 555–566

285. Yun CW & Lee SH. 'The roles of autophagy in cancer.' International Journal of Molecular Sciences 19 (2018) 3466

286. He C, Sumpter Jr. R & Levine B. 'Exercise induces autophagy in peripheral tissues and in the brain.' Autophagy 8 (2012) 1548–1551

287. Chauhan AK & Mallick BN. 'Association between autophagy and rapid eye movement sleep loss-associated neurodegenerative and patho-physio-behavioral changes.' Sleep Medicine 63 (2019) 29–37

288. Li Y et al. 'Autophagy Triggered by Oxidative Stress Appears to Be Mediated by the AKT/mTOR Signaling Pathway in the Liver of Sleep-Deprived Rats.' Oxidative Medicine and Cellular Longevity 2020 (2020)

289. de Groot S, Pijl H, van der Hoeven JJM & Kroep JR. 'Effects of short-term fasting on cancer treatment.' Journal of Experimental & Clinical Cancer Research 38 (2019) 209

290. William A. 'About Anthony William' (2020). Retrieved from https://www.medicalmedium.com/medical-medium-about-anthony-william (accessed Oct 2020)

291. William A. *Celery Juice* (Hay House, 2019)

292. Smith-Spangler C et al. 'Are organic foods safer or healthier than conventional alternatives? A systematic review.' Annals of Internal Medicine 157 (2012) 348–366

293. Baudry J et al. 'Association of frequency of organic food consumption with cancer risk: Findings from the NutriNet-Santé prospective cohort study.' JAMA Internal Medicine 178 (2018) 1597–1606

294. Heidary F, Rahimi A & Gharebaghi R. 'Poverty as a risk factor in human cancers.' Iranian Journal of Public Health 42 (2013) 341–343

295. Vohra J, Marmot MG, Bauld L & Hiatt RA. 'Socioeconomic position in childhood and cancer in adulthood: a rapid-review.' Journal of Epidemiology and Community Health 70 (2016) 629–634

296. Bradbury KE et al. 'Organic food consumption and the incidence of cancer in a large prospective study of women in the United Kingdom.' British Journal of Cancer 110 (2014) 2321–2326

297. Ames BN, Profet M & Gold LS. 'Dietary pesticides (99.99% all natural).' Proceedings of the National Academy of Sciences 87 (1990) 7777–7781

298. Messina M. 'Soy and health update: evaluation of the clinical and epidemiologic literature.' Nutrients 8 (2016) 754

299. Ju YH et al. 'Physiological concentrations of dietary genistein dose-dependently stimulate growth of estrogen-dependent human breast cancer (MCF-7) tumors implanted in athymic nude mice.' The Journal of Nutrition 131 (2001) 2957–2962

300. Setchell KDR et al. 'Soy isoflavone phase II metabolism differs between rodents and humans: implications for the effect on breast cancer risk.' The American Journal of Clinical Nutrition 94 (2011) 1284–1294

301. Ziaei S & Halaby R. 'Dietary isoflavones and breast cancer risk.' Medicines 4 (2017) 18

302. Hamilton-Reeves JM et al. 'Clinical studies show no effects of soy protein or isoflavones on reproductive hormones in men: results of a meta-analysis.' Fertility and Sterility 94 (2010) 997–1007

303. Storhaug CL, Fosse SK & Fadnes LT. 'Country, regional, and global estimates for lactose malabsorption in adults: a systematic review and meta-analysis.' The Lancet Gastroenterology & Hepatology 2 (2017) 738–746

304. Gambert I & Linné T. 'From Rice Eaters to Soy Boys: Race, Gender, and Tropes of "Plant Food Masculinity".' Animal Studies Journal 7 (2018) 129–179

305. Willhite CC et al. 'Systematic review of potential health risks posed by pharmaceutical, occupational and consumer exposures to metallic and nanoscale aluminum, aluminum oxides, aluminum hydroxide and its soluble salts.' Critical Reviews in Toxicology 44 (2014) 1–80

306. Lee AHS. 'Why is carcinoma of the breast more frequent in the upper outer quadrant? A case series based on needle core biopsy diagnoses.' The Breast 14 (2005) 151–152

307. Ellsworth DL et al. 'Outer breast quadrants demonstrate increased levels of genomic instability.' Annals of Surgical Oncology 11 (2004) 861–868

308. Flarend R, Bin T, Elmore D & Hem SL. 'A preliminary study of the dermal absorption of aluminium from antiperspirants using aluminium-26.' Food and Chemical Toxicology 39 (2001) 163–168

309. Schoenfeld JD & Ioannidis JPA. 'Is everything we eat associated with cancer? A systematic cookbook review.' The American Journal of Clinical Nutrition 97 (2013) 127–134

310. Penn State. 'Reduce Calories, Stave Off Hunger With Water-Rich Foods – Not Water' (1999). Retrieved from https://www.sciencedaily.com/releases/1999/09/990928074750.htm (accessed Dec 2020)

311. Tribole E & Resch E. *Intuitive Eating, 4th Edition* (St. Martin's Essentials, 2020)

312. Van Dyke N & Drinkwater EJ. 'Relationships between intuitive eating and health indicators: literature review.' Public Health Nutrition 17 (2014) 1757–1766

313. Bégin C et al. 'Eating-Related and Psychological Outcomes of Health at Every Size Intervention in Health and Social Services Centers Across the Province of Québec.' American Journal of Health Promotion 33 (2019) 248–258

Acknowledgements

It sounds obvious in retrospect, but writing a book was so much harder than I thought it would be. Don't get me wrong, I absolutely loved it, but can I do the next one *after* we're all done with surviving through a global pandemic?

To my beautiful partner Claire. Thank you so much for your continued patience and understanding, not only with the months I spent writing this book, but with my foray into social media that kicked all of this off. I love you.

My family, specifically my mother. If it wasn't for you, I wouldn't be anywhere near as well put together as I think I am today. I'm incredibly grateful for who you are. Chris and Peter Cason – I seem to remember promising you both that when we got a puppy you wouldn't end up doing all the walks . . . and then the exact opposite happened! Thank you for being so gracious about it.

To Alan Flanagan, Lindo Bacon and Pixie Turner for taking the time to review and offer much needed feedback on the manuscript. Your opinions and advice were invaluable, and I appreciate all of you.

To my incredibly supportive friends who are never afraid to challenge and put me in my place. You know who you are.

The entire team at Vermilion, with particular thanks to my editing duo, Emma Owen and Leah Feltham, and my copy editor Becky Alexander. I want to apologise profusely for my poor grasp on what it means when I say I'll send it 'later today'. Thank you for all your hard work and patience.

To Max Parker, for being my first ever hype man during initial publisher meetings. To my manager Andrew Selby and the rest of the team at 84world for continuing to represent me despite my unorthodox attitude when it comes to being an influencer.

To those on social media who send me messages of support on a regular basis. You remind me why I'm doing this when I want to pack it all in. Please don't stop.

Finally, to all those I have learned and benefited from in the HAES space. I'd have no idea what I was doing without the work of those with far less privilege who had so much to lose by speaking out. I don't take that for granted.

INDEX